Get Through

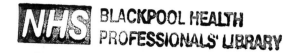
MRCGP: Oral and Video Modules

Get Through
MRCGP: Oral and Video Modules

Una Coales BA (Hons) MD FRCS FRCSOto DRCOG DFFP MRCGP
GP, London, UK

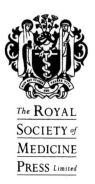

The ROYAL
SOCIETY *of*
MEDICINE
PRESS *Limited*

© 2004 Royal Society of Medicine Ltd

Reprinted 2006

Published by the Royal Society of Medicine Press Ltd
1 Wimpole Street, London W1G 0AE, UK
Tel: +44 (0)20 7290 2921
Fax: +44 (0)20 7290 2929
E-mail: publishing@rsm.ac.uk
Website: www.rsmpress.co.uk

British Library Cataloging in Publication Data
A catalogue record for this book is available from the British Library

ISBN: 1-85315-593-4

Distribution in Europe and Rest of the World:

Marston Book Services Ltd
PO Box 269
Abingdon
Oxon OX14 4YN, UK
Tel: +44 (0)1235 465500
Fax: +44 (0)1235 465666

Distribution in USA and Canada:

Royal Society of Medicine Press Ltd
c/o JAMCO Distribution Inc
1401 Lakeway Drive
Lewisville, TX 75057, USA
Tel: +1 800 538 1287
Fax: +1 972 353 1303
E-mail: jamco@majors.com

Distribution in Australia and New Zealand:

Elsevier Australia
30–52 Smidmore Street
Marrikville NSW 2204, Australia
Tel: +61 2 9517 8999
Fax: +61 2 9517 2249
E-mail: service@elsevier.com.au

Phototypeset by Phoenix Photosetting, Chatham, Kent
Printed in the UK by Bell & Bain, Glasgow, UK

Contents

Preface

This book accompanies *Get Through MRCGP: New MCQ Module* and covers both the viva and new 2004 video components of the MRCGP exam. As I have been approached by numerous registrars seeking advice on how to pass these components, I have decided to incorporate my material into this handy book. To pass the viva module, the candidate must be aware that the bank of questions on which the examiners rely is based on a 4×3 grid of 12 possible topics. This book covers that grid and gives numerous examples of questions that have been asked. To pass the video module, the candidate should understand the 14 performance criteria (PCs) that the examiners are looking for and ensure these are clearly demonstrated in the videotaped consultations. Not only do I give tips on how to pass the video module, but I have also included the actual transcript from all my 11 videotaped consultations, of which the first seven were used for the MRCGP exam and passed, and how I completed the video logbook as a guide to candidates.

Una Coales

UFCMD@aol.com

Recommended texts and references

Birtwhistle J et al. (2002) Oxford Handbook of General Practice. Oxford: Oxford University Press

Chana N et al. (2001) An Insider's Guide to the Oral Exam. Oxford: Radcliffe Medical Press

Coales U. (2003) Get Through MRCGP: New MCQ Module. London: The Royal Society of Medicine Press Ltd.

Health and Safety Commission (1999) Management of health and safety at work. Approved code of practice and guidance, HSE books

Health and Safety Commission (1995) A guide to the reporting of injuries, diseases and dangerous occurrences regulations 1995, HSE books

Kilburn J. (2001) Answer Plans for the MRCGP. Oxford: Bio Scientific Publishers Ltd.

Neighhbour R. (2002) The Inner Consultation. Berkshire: Librapharm Ltd.

Palmer KT. (2001) Notes for the MRCGP, 3rd edn. Oxford: Blackwell Science Ltd.

The Royal College of General Practitioners (2003) MRCGP Video Assessment of Consulting Skills Workbook and Instructions

1. MRCGP oral module

You will arrive at the Royal College, register, be given a name sticker and be asked to wait in the sitting room, which offers tea, coffee, and water. The convener will ask one group at a time to follow him up the stairs to the examining rooms for the first of the 20-minute examinations. The oral consists of two separate 20-minute examinations. You will be asked to sit at a table of two examiners, who will take 10-minute turns to ask you questions. One marks while the other examines you. When the bell goes, you will be directed to another table or room for the second of the 20-minute examinations and two new examiners. At the sound of the next bell, you will be asked to leave. The oral examination will be over.

It is important that you realize that the marking starts subconsciously when you enter the room! You should be dressed in a suit (trouser suits are fine for women if preferred). Confidently approach the examiners and offer to shake their hands. Introduce yourself and they will introduce themselves also. Be seen to be making a conscious effort to learn their names, i.e. repeat out loud the names on the name-cards on the table. They will ask you how you got to the college. Be polite and smile. It is not unusual for candidates to experience the fight or flight reaction and freeze. If your voice starts feeling tight, exhale and then take a deep breath. You will notice now that your ability to talk has returned.

Beware, as you will fail if you are seen to fidget, speak too softly or too slowly, leave long gaps between answering questions or have few options to offer the examiners when questioned. I have this on authority from an examiner!

Examiners are given the same grid of questions, so you may be asked the same topics at both tables. Take advantage of this second opportunity to get it right! The marking grid consists of a 4×3 table (Table 1). On the left side, the four topics covered include care of patients, working with colleagues, society, and personal responsibility. On the top of the grid are the headings communication, professional values, and personal and professional growth. For instance, examiners compose questions by combining a topic on the left side of the grid with one of the three headings. One example would be asking a question regarding communication and care of patients, i.e. Describe examples of nonverbal and verbal communication? How do you know if the consultation is going well?

If you receive a rapid fire of questions, you are doing well. They will seem to push you but don't be alarmed, as you will have passed by then. If you do not know the answer, say so, which will allow the examiner to move on, unless he is being particularly difficult. If you are asked what you would do in a given situation, always answer, 'I would ...' and not 'my trainer would ...' or 'I have heard that ...' or 'I have read that ...'. Ooze confidence! Speak clearly and succinctly. You may realize that under pressure, you will speak at twice your normal rate. Slow down! Practice in front of a mirror or with a friend. You should appear natural and calm.

This section gives specific questions that have been asked and examples of how to answer these questions. Think grid and in which box the examiner wants to give you marks, when you answer the question. This will help you focus and give him the answer he wants to hear. I have managed to cover a vast number of popular questions, so you should not be taken by surprise and should be able to approach the examiners with full confidence and expect to pass the oral!

Table I Oral module marking grid

	Communication	Professional values	Personal and professional growth
Care of patients	Breaking bad news (empathy) Effective information transfer (motivation) Consultation models Communication with adolescents (verbal and nonverbal) Translators	Expensive drugs Flexibility and tolerance Medicolegal issues Morality and ethics Patient autonomy Revalidation Terminal care	Audit EBM Negotiating change Patients as educators Self-appraisal Which patients cause stress
Working with colleagues	Complaints Practice meetings Staff appraisal Teaching medical students Teamwork	Clinical guidelines Community pharmacists Sick doctors	Access Appraisal Away days Management of burnout NHS Direct Stress awareness Underperformance
Society	Health promotion Communication with the media Practice leaflets Teenage health	Euthanasia Gatekeeping role/cost Rationing/cost	Death of a partner Generalists New drugs Out-of-hours care Quality of care
Personal responsibility	Aggressive patients Asylum seekers Effective consulting Heart-sink patients	Advance directives Gifts Whistleblowing	Change and change management CME Hazards of GP Mentoring Study leave Uncertainty

Marking of the oral module

Candidates are graded on each topic on a scale of 1–9. The nine marks range from 'outstanding', 'excellent', 'good', 'satisfactory', 'bare pass', 'not adequate', 'unsatisfactory', 'poor', to 'dangerous'. Your four examiners then meet to determine the overall mark for the oral, an aggregate of the four marks given during the two oral exams. They are only permitted to round up.

1. What is risk management? (Personal responsibility, care of patients, working with colleagues, society/professional values)

Risk management evolved from the Health and Safety at Work Act of 1974. In 1999, the Health and Safety Commission (HSC) approved the code of practice entitled the management of health and safety at work. This regulation requires all employers to assess the risks to workers and any others who may be affected by their work or business. All employers should carry out a systematic general examination of the effect of their undertaking, their work activities and the condition of the premises.

Therefore risk management involves firstly, identifying potential hazards (something with the potential to cause harm) to health and safety to any person arising out of, or in connection with, work or the conduct of their undertaking. It should identify how the risks arise and how they impact on those affected. Secondly, make an assessment of the risk to the patient, to the doctor, to the practice and to society as a whole. Risk is defined as the likelihood of potential harm from that hazard being realised. Thirdly, significant findings should be recorded in writing and reviewed and revised regularly. This includes a significant event audit (SEA) and adverse incident reporting (AIR).

An easy pneumonic is Bransford and Stein's (1984) IDEAL – identify, define, explore, act, look back (reassess).

Risk to the patient

Assessing the risk to the patient includes:

1. Assessing the premises of the surgery:

   - Ensure clear access to the building.

   - Ensure that the waiting room is clear of hazards. A patient may sue if he slips on a wet floor. Ensure that the consulting room is safe. For example, the sharps bin should not be placed within reach of a child. A claim was made against a GP who was found to be negligent after a child placed his hand in a sharps bin while the GP was examining the mother.

2. A doctor whose own health is poor has an obligation to cooperate with the General Medical Council's (GMC's) health procedures.

Risk to the doctor of litigation

The Medical Defence Union (MDU) have issued tips under the heading Risk Management Advice to the Doctor to Avoid Litigation:

- Risk of complaints and claims often result from failure to carry out an adequate examination of a patient. This includes taking a proper history, conducting the appropriate physical examination and carrying out baseline investigations.
- Maintain full and accurate records.
- Ensure good communication between the doctor and patient to develop effective clinical care and establish good trust.
- A perceived uncaring attitude may motivate a complainant to pursue a claim.
- Do not breach confidentiality. If you do, justify your actions.
- Decisions regarding do not resuscitate (DNR) orders should be made only after discussion with the patient and/or relatives, have consultant approval and be documented in the clinical notes.
- A doctor who accepts to provide a medicolegal report should do so within a reasonable time scale.
- Doctors have an obligation to act if they believe that patient care is likely to be compromised by the conduct, performance or health of the other healthcare professionals. They must have sufficient grounds for raising concerns and be prepared to back up their allegations with more detailed observations where appropriate.
- Allegations of indecent assault may be avoided if the doctor gives a detailed explanation of the exam and why it is necessary. Document that you have asked the patient whether he or she would like a chaperone if performing an intimate exam (breast, per vagina [PV], or per rectum [PR]).
- Personal relationships (emotional or sexual) with patients are not advised, even after the clinical relationship has ended to avoid allegations of use of professional position to influence or take advantage of someone in a vulnerable position.
- Professional competence must be maintained and renewed on a lifelong basis to ensure a good standard of care and practice.

Risk to doctor of burnout, violent patients, exposure to blood or body fluids, etc.

Give the examiner as many examples of categories as you can. Go into detail if asked.

Risk to the practice

All employees are advised by law to read the practice's guidelines to health and safety in the workplace. If an accident occurs in the workplace and the employee is not aware of these guidelines, the employer is not liable.

Accidents may involve patients and potential hazards should be identified and removed.

Risk to society

This may cover sectioning of a patient who is at risk to self or to society under the Mental Health Act of 1983.

Section 2 admits for compulsory admission of a patient to hospital for assessment of patient for up to 28 days and requires two doctors (one approved under section 12 and one GP).

Section 3 admits for compulsory admission to hospital for treatment up to 6 months and requires a diagnosis and two doctors (one approved under section 23 and one GP).

Section 4 admits for compulsory admission to hospital as an 'urgent necessity' for 72 hours and requires one doctor who has seen the patient within the last 24 hours and one social worker or nearest relative.

Section 5 allows a doctor or nominated deputy (nurse) to detain an inpatient for 72 hours in an emergency only and requires that a psychiatrist be contacted as soon as can be arranged.

Section 135 gives police the right of entry into premises to remove a person to a place of safety under a magistrate's warrant.

Section 136 gives police the right to remove a person from a public place to a place of safety for 72 hours to allow a medical examination.

How do you conduct a significant event analysis?

You should:

- Pre-arrange a meeting and ensure all staff involved in the event are present.
- Set ground rules.
- Identify the facts and address the issues raised.
- Identify what went well and what went badly.
- Discuss what improvement might be made.
- Agree on what action to take.
- Identify any new resources or skills which are needed.
- Agree on when and how the changes will be evaluated.

2. What is fitness to practice? List the seven codes of good medical practice. (Professional values/care of patients, working with colleagues, personal responsibility)

Obtain a free copy of the *Good Medical Practice* booklet from the General Medical Council and absorb this short 19-page booklet. In short, the seven codes of practice are:

1. Providing good clinical care.
2. Maintaining good medical practice – keeping up to date, maintaining your performance.
3. Teaching and training, appraising and assessing.
4. Relationships with patients – obtaining consent, respecting confidentiality, maintaining trust, good communication.
5. Working with colleagues – treat colleagues fairly, working in teams, with a team leader, sharing information, delegation and referral.
6. Probity – providing information regarding your services, writing reports, giving evidence, signing documents, research, financial and commercial dealings, conflicts of interest.
7. Your health – if your health may put patients at risk.

Commit them to memory, and be able to recite them smoothly.

3. How would you recognise stress in yourself? (Personal and professional growth/care of patients)

There are four stages to burnout:

1. Overwork
2. Frustration
3. Resentment
4. Depression.

Signs of stress/burnout include increased irritability/anger with family and colleagues, fatigue, accident-proneness, depression, alcohol/drug abuse, low self-esteem, low productivity, poor time-keeping, inefficiency, increased sick leave, increased mistakes, relationship problems, poor decision making, and depersonalisation (treating patients as objects). Family and colleagues may notice signs and make you aware.

Maslach's burnout inventory includes emotional exhaustion, depersonalisation and reduced levels of achievement).

Factors contributing to burnout include inappropriate demands, unsociable hours, heart-sink patients, etc.)

The solution is good time management, taking frequent breaks, retaining a good sense of humour, setting realistic goals, exercise/hobbies, support from colleagues, learning assertiveness skills, organisational skills, etc.

Maintain Sense of humor; good views outside window
Interest outside of medicine
Exercise
Prioritising
Having a good mean.
Talking to Peers.
Relaxation techniques
Confident, Remain flexible, being able to ask for help
ability to say no.
Guilt free delegations.

4A. How do you know if the consultation is going well? Going poorly? And why?

4B. What can you do to elicit the patient's hidden agenda? (Communication/care of patients)

Signs that the consultation is going well

These include:

- Non-verbal cues, i.e. body language – the patient is smiling, nodding, maintaining good eye contact, their body is turned towards you, and the patient shakes your hand at the end of the consultation.

- Verbal cues – the patient shows understanding verbally, thanks you, asks to see you in particular in the future, asks you how long you will be staying at the practice.

Signs that the consultation is going poorly

- Non-verbal cues – the patient is fidgeting in his chair, avoids eye contact, has their body turned away from you, expresses discontent on his face, stands up and starts pacing, refuses to leave the room.

- Verbal cues – the patient continues to list more problems that need addressing ('by the way ...'), as he or she does not feel as though the initial needs were met. The patient raises his voice, changes the tone of his voice, challenges you, undermines your confidence, becomes aggressive, asks to see the manager, asks to see another doctor, tells you he is unhappy, declares that he will put in a complaint, etc.

Reasons consultations become dysfunctional

- Doctor – running late, does not have the notes, has preconceived perceptions of patient, fails to uncover the real reason for the patient's visit
- Patient – a language barrier, noisy children present in the room, illiteracy, too unwell to communicate, excessive anxiety, intoxicated.
- External – constant interruptions by phone or at the door, noisy waiting room.

Communication techniques

1. Non-verbal – maintain good eye contact, uncross arms and legs, try not to focus your attention on the monitor or the set of notes in front of you, give full attention to the patient (furrow eyebrows and squint, and turn chair to face patient), use of touch.
2. Verbal – using communication models, say 'Is there anything else?', and use the SCORES method:
   - Silence
   - Clarify
   - Open-ended questions
   - Reflecting back
   - Empathic response
   - Summarise

Tate's strategy for a successful consultation

1. Why has the patient come?
2. Is this the real reason? Is there anything else?
3. Have I explored any underlying thoughts?
4. Is there an underlying reason?
5. Have I understood the thoughts and reasons?
6. Have I given appropriate responses?
7. Have we got a happy patient and a happy doctor?

5. What is your favourite consultation model and why? (Communication/care of patients)

The correct answer is Roger Neighbour's The Inner Consultation, 1987. You may answer Pendleton's The Consultation, An Approach to Learning and Teaching, 1984, but it is less popular and you will end up defending your choice.

Roger's five checklist stages are:

1. **Connecting** – establishing rapport with the patient. This refers to rapport building and may include skills such as acceptance set, curtain raiser/opening gambit, internal search, matching, NLP, and speech censoring. Suffice it to say, if you reply with just my first sentence you will gain points.

2. **Summarising** – getting to the point of why the patient has come, using skills of eliciting to discover their ideas, concerns and expectations (ICE) and summarising back to the patient. The listening and eliciting skills include the patient is right to start with, explain why you are asking, be facilitative and encouraging (with open-ended questions, statements, my friend John), echoing and checking.

3. **Handing over** – doctors and patients' agenda agreed. Skills include negotiating, influencing (doctor's apostolic function) and gift-wrapping ('You don't need those nasty antibiotics this time').

4. **Safety-netting** – 'What if?' predicting skills – what would the doctor do in each case.

5. **Housekeeping** – Taking care of yourself – Am I in good enough shape for the next patient? Get up and stretch, have a cup of coffee, go to the loo.

Whichever one of Roger's checklists you prefer, don't forget to give a reason why. 'I like his safety-netting tip, as it allows me to deal with uncertainty…' The examiners want you to be able to incorporate learning points into your consultation, not just recite a model back to them. However the examiner may turn around and ask you to discuss Pendleton's model, so below I have given you a summary of all the consultation models to have at your disposal.

1984 Pendleton's The Consultation, An Approach to Learning and Teaching

The seven tasks to an ideal consultation are:

1. To define the reason for the patient's attendance, including:
   - The nature and history of the problem
   - Their cause
   - The patient's ideas, concerns and expectations
   - The effects of their problems
2. To consider other problems:
   - At-risk factors
   - Continuing problems
3. To choose with the patient an appropriate action for each problem.
4. To achieve a shared understanding of the problem with the patient.
5. To involve the patient in the management plan and encourage him to accept appropriate responsibility.
6. To use time and resources appropriately:
   - In the consultation
   - In the long term
7. To establish or maintain a relationship with the patient that helps to achieve the other tasks.

1981 Helman's Folk Model

Cecil Helman is a medical anthropologist and suggests that a patient with a problem comes to a doctor seeking answers to six questions:

1. What has happened?
2. Why has this happened?
3. Why to me?
4. Why now?
5. What would happen if nothing was done about it?
6. What should I do about or whom should I consult for further help?

1979 Stott and Davis

A	B
Management of presenting problems	Modification of help-seeking behaviours
C	D
Management of continuing problems	Opportunistic health promotion

TVO5515

1976 Byrne and Long's Doctors Talking to Patient

A study of 2500 audio-taped consultations led to a description of six phases, which occur in a consultation:

1. The doctor establishes a relationship with the patient.
2. The doctor either attempts to discover or actually discovers the reason for the patient's attendance.
3. The doctor conducts a verbal or physical examination, or both.
4. The doctor, or the doctor and the patient, or the patient considers the condition.
5. The doctor and occasionally the patient details treatment or further investigation.
6. The consultation is terminated, usually by the doctor.

1975 John Heron's Six Category Intervention Analysis

Heron is a humanist psychologist who described the behaviour of health professionals or the interventions of a doctor as one of six interventions:

1. Prescriptive – giving advice or instructions; being critical or directive.
2. Informative – imparting new knowledge, instructing or interpreting.
3. Confrontational – challenging a restrictive attitude or behaviour; giving direct feedback within a caring context.
4. Cathartic – seeking to release emotion in the form of weeping, laughter, trembling or anger.
5. Catalytic – encouraging the patient to discover and explore his own latent thoughts and feelings.
6. Supportive – offering comfort and approval; affirming the patient's intrinsic value.

1966 Eric Berne's Games People Play

- **Transactional Analysis** – he classifies the states of mind as parent, adult and child and that an individual has a given repertoire of behaviour corresponding to this state of mind.
- **The Child** – spontaneous or dependent. Many GP consultations are conducted between a parental doctor and a child-like patient and may not be in the best interests of the patient. The doctor should be aware of transactional analysis and be flexible enough to change his repertoire to avoid consultations degenerating into the games people play.
- **The Adult** – this logical ego state is concerned with problem solving, taking in data and processing, and storing knowledge and skills.

- **The Parent** – critical or caring, nurturing or controlling. The transactions during consultations may be complimentary, crossed or ulterior.

1957 Balint's The Doctor, His Patient and the Illness

The three main themes are: (1) psychological problems are often manifested physically and physical disease causes psychological problems, (2) doctors have feelings too and these feelings can impact on the consultation process, and (3) doctors can be trained in a limited way to be more sensitive to what is going on in the patient's mind.

Balintian concepts:

1. The Doctor as a Drug.

2. The Child as the Presenting Complaint – ticket of entry.

3. Elimination by Appropriate Physical Examination.

4. Collusion of Anonymity – nobody taking final responsibility for the patient.

5. The Flash – the real reason for attendance is made apparent to both the doctor and the patient.

6. The Mutual Investment Company – the patient presents with episodic offers of both physical and psychological problems in a long relationship.

6. If a partner requests 5 weeks' study leave to take a residential creative writing course, how does that impact on the practice? (Personal responsibility/personal and professional growth)

There are issues for the partner's patients, his colleagues, the practice, society as a whole and for the partner in question.

Issues for his patients would be loss of continuity of care if he is absent for 5 weeks at a time.

Issues for his colleagues would be the time and expense involved to find a locum or to cover his work themselves. The partner should realise this would be a tremendous burden on the other partners, who would also question how a residential creative writing course would benefit the practice and may build resentment to this partner.

Issues for the practice include a reduction in manpower, loss of continuity of care for my patients, locum expenses, longer waiting time for appointments, etc.

The issue for society is that there is one less GP working to cover a list of 2400 patients per GP.

The issues for the partner in question are rationalising why he needs to take 5 weeks' study leave for a creative writing course. How would it benefit his personal and professional growth? Is it to relieve stress and reduce burnout, and perhaps help his emotional well-being? But he also has a personal responsibility to his patients, to the partners and to the practice. He would have to justify such a request and discuss the matter with all concerned at the practice.

- Can offer Sabbatical (unpaid leave)
- 1 week study leave.
- a soft way of leaving the practice.

7. How would you encourage more interest in general practice? (Society/communication)

This question explores different forms of communication with society. I would suggest encouraging awareness of general practice by using all the forms of media that are available nowadays. An ad in the local paper, a TV commercial, more information available to the public and to medical students on the Internet, an ad on the radio, open days at schools, medical schools, fliers in hospital lobbies or schools.

Personally, I think we should increase awareness with teenagers and with medical students by inviting them to spend a day with a GP. As of August 2004, it will be mandatory for all junior doctors to rotate through general practice as part of their foundation years.

8. What is a heart-sink patient? If one partner had many more heart-sink patients than the other partners, what does this mean? What is good about having heart-sink patients for you and for the practice? (It is not good). (Personal responsibility/communication)

According to Clarke and Croft, 1998 Critical Reading for the Reflective Practitioner, Balint defined heartsink as the feelings induced in a GP by patients' (frustration, hopelessness, inadequacy, irritation). Examples include frequent attenders, somatisers, patients with lists, dysfunctional consultations, etc.

In 1978, Groves, an American psychiatrist, classified 'hateful' patients into four stereotypes:

1. Dependent clinger – these patients will not take responsibility. The solution is to limit the number of investigations, referrals and have the patient see one doctor exclusively, if possible.

2. Entitled demander – a patient who consults more than the average 3.5 times per year, excessive demands, 'I know my rights!', dissatisfied with service provided. **Do not enter into a debate.** Simply, tell the patient that you are doing your best to ensure they get the best possible medical care.

3. Manipulative help rejector, i.e. an intravenous drug abuser (IVDA). Nothing has worked for this patient. The solution is to share their pessimism, by saying 'There may be no cure for your ailment,' or 'This treatment is not entirely curative.'

4. Self-destructive denier – is in denial of the risk factors, i.e. an alcoholic. The solution is to offer compassion.

In general, the solution to managing heart-sink patients is to have a more balanced and realistic view of the consultation:

1. Take control of the consultation.

2. Understand the patient's game.

3. Structure future consultations.

4. Encourage lists. Take the patient's list and inform them that they have booked a 10-minute consultation with you and for them to select the most important item and to rebook for the rest.

5. Say 'What do you think I can do to help you?', 'I don't know if medical science has an answer for you', or 'What is your reason for not changing or trying this option?'

6. Make sure they realise what their problem is – smoking, obesity etc. Don't let them leave their 'monkeys' on your shoulder or in your room. Hand responsibility back to the patient.

7. Set rules. Say 'I will see you in 6 weeks.' So they don't come back over and over.

8. Discuss the patient. Share the consultation with a partner.

Clark and Croft suggest the following approach when dealing with somatising patients:

1. Obtain a full history and don't forget to explore ICE, emotional issues, and psychosocial (family) issues.

2. Acknowledge the reality of the symptoms and their effects.

3. Broaden the agenda – give an honest feedback of the results of the exams, explain and reframe.

4. Make the link that psychological distress can cause physical symptoms and see if the explanation is accepted.

Why would one partner have more heart-sink patients than the others?

Matters paper suggests that the number of heart-sink patients one has is proportional to the degree of one's poor communication skills. Heart-sink patients tend to be found more in lower socioeconomic classes, where doctors have a high patient load, and are burnt out. The solution would be to lessen the patient load, suggest a communication course for the doctor, sit in with another partner, try to give insight to the doctor, etc.

(1) Can video-tape
(2) attend Course
(3) Read books on Communication skills.

9. What is the double-effect? (Personal responsibility, care of patients/professional values/society)

An example would be morphine, which has both a positive and negative effect. It decreases pain and yet is used to shorten life in the terminally ill. This question may lead to a talk on euthanasia.

If stuck on a topic you are not up-to-date with, use the following structure and cover the bullet points in an attempt to give a logical and plausible response:

Issues for the doctor (it is best to take a side – for/against euthanasia and why)

- Duty to act in the patient's best interest
- Beneficence – do no harm
- Own personal moral code or religious objections
- Non-judgemental care
- Awareness of current evidence/guidelines (model forms may be obtained from the Voluntary Euthanasia Society or the Terence Higgins Trust and are legally binding)
- Assessment of patient's motivation
- Need to sort out immediate clinical need
- Need to justify action
- Perceived pressure to support/oppose
- Uncertainty
- Shared care/seek advice from Medical Defence Union (MDU)
- Consent
- Conflicts of interest
- Good record keeping

Issues for the patient

- Patient's reasons for request
- Patient's concerns and expectations

- Patient's underlying, hidden agenda (emotional, medical needs)
- Fear of loss of autonomy and dignity
- Explore patient's belief regarding his own health
- Embarassment and fears
- Patient's social and family background
- Cultural beliefs
- Relevant life events
- Impaired ability to cope
- Assess available support
- Assess patient's knowledge and understanding
- Patient must be involved in all plans and decisions
- Awareness of the dangers
- Advance directives/living wills – ensure that the wishes of a competent patient are considered when informed consent can no longer be obtained to refuse specific treatment. It requires a fully informed patient, review every 5 years, and asks the patient to inform the relatives. The GP's role is as an advisor or repository. Guidance may be obtained from the British Medical Association (BMA) Ethics Division.

Issues for the practice

- Agreed practice guidelines/policy

Legal and ethical issues

- Personal ethics
- Informed consent
- Consult BMA, General Medical Council (GMC) and MDU.

Wider issues

- Awareness of new treatments

I echo the voice of our chairman Prof. Mayur Lakhani" in his statement to Press " Systems that are in place are adequate & doctors act in pt's best interest".

Netherlands, Belgium, State of Oregon in America → assisted dying allowed

Assisted dying in terminally ill → Lord Joffe.

21

10. A patient took a friend's prescriptive drug by mistake and says it works wonders for her osteoarthritis (OA). She is now adamant she wants more bendrofluazide for OA. What are the issues? (Care of patients, personal responsibility/ professional values). Discuss the issues for you, the patient, the practice and wider issues. Use the previous answer as a guide to structure. Ensure your answer addresses the ethical issues

Mention Beauchamp and Childress: benevolence, nonmaleficence, duty of care.

Incorporate the five components of ethics into your answer:

1. Autonomy

2. Beneficence (doing good)

3. Concern/confidentiality

4. Do no harm

5. Equity.

Outline your clinical management

- Bower and Bower model – DESC – describe, explain 'makes me concerned', specify one change in the future, consequences (benefits – gift-wrapping)

- Documentation

- Express your self-awareness.

- Discuss the wider issues for the practice and society.

11. How would you conduct a staff appraisal? How would you acknowledge and build morale? (Communication/working with colleagues)

Definition

Appraisal is a positive process to give feedback on someone's past performance, to chart their continuing progress and to identify needs and should be performed annually. Appraisal for GPs specifically covers the headings of good clinical care, maintaining good medical practice, relationships with patients, working with colleagues, teaching and training, probity and health and may be adapted for any health professional or employee in your practice.

Models

Berne's Transactional Analytic Format

The GP assumes the parental role, is in an ego state, and acknowledges the employee as an adult and not a child.

I would use both verbal and non-verbal forms of communication. I would encourage her to express her views with open-ended questions, clarify what she has said by repeating back to her, and summarise the conversation. Non-verbal techniques include the use of silence, showing empathy, and the use of non-threatening body language. I would wish to hand over responsibility back to her with regards to addressing her own mutually agreed future needs.

Pendleton's Rules for Feedback

The assessor would say:

- 'You tell me what has been good about the past year?'
- 'Then I tell you what I think has been good.'
- 'Is there anything you could have done better?'
- 'Well I've noticed this could be better.'

Then would:

- Agree together with the employee on what can be done in future.

Review an employee's performance, goals and development.

Can not fail appraisal.

Blake and Maslow's Humanistic Theory

'A human being is a motivated organism within an effective, cohesive and structured organisation. Leadership is an attempt to direct and motivate people and arrange the organisation effectively to support the followers' efforts and increase their sense of personal worth.'

'I would use positive reinforcement, performance-related pay, say or write 'Thank you', arrange practice Christmas parties, etc.'

To score merit points, don't forget to drop names such as Pendleton, Berne, Neighbour or Blake and Maslow.

1st Confirm death, inform the Coroner.

to relatives :- extremely empathetic

Practice :- SEA.

District nurse should adjust syringe driver.

12. Scenario: You make a home visit and realise that the patient's relative has run a morphine driver over 8 hours and not 24 hours by mistake, and now the patient is dead. What are the issues? (Professional values, care of patients)

The issues for the patient's family are the need to organize burial and therefore need for death certificate, immediate grief reaction/bereavement (denial, anger, guilt, depression).

In helping the family deal with bereavement I will listen and allow them to express their grief. I am ultimately a witness to this family death. I will facilitate them to take the actions they need to take with regards to the funeral. I will personally arrange bereavement visits to the family. I would give them a copy of *What to do After a Death*, a booklet issued by the DSS office.

The issues for the doctor are any uncertainty with regard to the medicolegal issues, empathy for the family and acknowledgement of my own grief at the loss of a well-known patient. I would debrief with colleagues. I would be aware that all death certificates I issue may be under scrutiny so I must be aware of the correct medicolegal requirements and also keep a register of deaths in the practice.

The issues for the practice are accurate documentation and any medicolegal issues covered later.

The medicolegal issues for society require accurate documentation and attendance to strict medicolegal requirements. Inform the coroner's office. If it is out-of-hours, contact the police station and ask for the coroner's officer or leave a message and they will ring you back. A coroner's officer is usually a retired police officer. Explain to the family that the coroner's officer will be in touch and the need for an autopsy.

The coroner will tell you whether he will issue the death certificate or advise you to. Without a death certificate documenting the cause of death, no-one may be cremated or buried. A death certificate is also required to stop pension payments and bill requests.

Deaths that should be reported to a coroner are:

- Death of a patient not seen by a doctor within the last 14 days

- Death occurring within 24 hours of an operation or administration of anaesthetic

- Death related to industrial disease, an industrial accident or road traffic accident (RTA)
- Death in prison or in police custody
- When there has been an accidental injury within the last year
- When there is an unknown cause of death
- In an unnatural, violent or suspicious death (accidents, drug-related, hypothermia, neglect by others, pneumonia following a fractured neck of femur, secondary to abortion, self-neglect, or suicide).

Do not touch or move anything at the scene. Confirm death of the patient and then call the police. The coroner may ask you for a report, so make detailed notes of everything you observe as you may also be called to give evidence. There is no issue of confidentiality when reporting to the coroner. The coroner's officer will tell you when the body may be removed for a funeral director, who is usually on-call 24 hours a day.

13. What is a practice development plan? (Personal and professional growth/ personal responsibility, working with colleagues)

Definition

Where are we now? Where do we want to be? How are we going to get there? How will we know when we have arrived there? This question is about change management.

Pre-meeting agenda

Prioritise

Arrange a locum to cover for you on the study day.

Designate a chairman

Decide who will attend and notify? (all healthcare professionals and practice staff).

Specifics

Where are we now?

1. Look at the practice area (demographics, goals – targets, teaching).
2. Practice ethos – aims, high quality of care, good incentives to local community.
3. Staffing – recruitment, retention, audit, teaching, strengths/weaknesses.
4. Premises – inadequate to deliver service.
5. Look at what we have achieved – each team member to perform a SWOT analysis (strengths, weaknesses, opportunities, and threats).

Where are we going?

1. Set goals, share goals and seek agreement – training practice growth to provide service to 7000–8000 patients, health improvement plan (HIMP), sexual health for teenagers, tackle low-birthweight babies), start morning breakfast club at local schools, etc.

2. Agree priorities.

3. Construct a strategy for the process of change – plan to sell our ideas to the local primary care team (PCT) in return for support of our needs.

4. Define the criteria for success or failure and the time scale.

How are we going to get there?

1. Clarify current resources – budget, funding.

2. Identify obstacles – PCT.

3. Identify helpful factors – volunteers, community support.

4. Conduct a SWOT analysis.

5. Select a team leader who will facilitate and a way to monitor change within an agreed timescale.

6. Delegate tasks.

7. Instigate change.

How will we know when we have arrived?

1. Assess the endpoint.

2. Evaluate the process.

3. Identify potential learning needs.

4. Acknowledge success.

14. How do you go about telling an employee that you are making them redundant? (Communication/care of patients)

What the examiner is after, is how you go about **breaking bad news**. I would use the Pendleton model for breaking bad news or Berne's model of transactional analysis and take on the caring parent to child role.

Whichever model you choose, make sure you cover the following key points:

1. Preparation for the meeting:

   Practice manager should be present to take minutes.

   - Know the facts.
   - Arrange for privacy without possible interruptions. Choose the right moment.
   - Set time boundaries. *fix a warning shot.*
   - Consider who should be present.

2. What is known?

   - Establish what the employee (patient) knows and wants to know. Check understanding.
   - Observe the employee's (patient's) manner, expression, beliefs, both verbal and non-verbal cues.

3. Is more information wanted?

   - What else does the employee (patient) want to know?

4. Allow for denial.

   - Establish how the employee (patient) is feeling now.

5. Sharing the information

   - Be clear and simple. Avoid jargon.
   - Give warning shots. Give information in small portions.
   - Keep checking for understanding and concerns.
   - Be gentle.
   - Avoid assumptions.
   - Know when to stop.

6. Elicit concerns.

What are the main concerns now? Respond to the employee's (patient's) feelings.

- Say 'Have you been surprised by what I have said?, How are you feeling?'
- Identify and acknowledge the employee's (patient's) feelings.
- Use prompts – 'Is there anything you are worried about? Is there anything else you would like to ask me?'
- Listen and give them time to phrase their questions.
- Good listening will make the employee (patient) feel heard and understood.

7. Summary and plan:

- Summarise concerns but be positive. Foster hope.
- Outline a future management plan, if appropriate.
- Check employee's (patient's) understanding again. Say 'Is all this making sense?'

8. Make a contract for further contact.

- Arrange a follow-up meeting and ensure support.

9. Ensure others are informed of what was said.

- Inform the practice team so that everyone is aware.
- Keep a record of the event.

15. Should there be occupational health for doctors? (Personal responsibility/professional values)

This question is an indirect method of asking about burnout, stress management, risk to doctor's health from patients, and self-awareness. These topics have been addressed earlier.

16. How do you keep your skills up-to-date? (Personal responsibility/personal growth)

Be honest! I have a personal development folder. I read the abstracts from the *British Medical Journal* and select interesting articles to read. I find the *British Journal of General Practice* tedious. I take courses that have PGEA approval or CME points. I have started the appraisal process. I use patient's unmet needs (PUNS) and doctor's educational needs (DENS) as a good learning tool:

1. Personal development plan/accreditation of personal development (APD), maintain an educational portfolio (notes, handouts, articles, audits, completed activities, reflections, evaluations etc.)

2. Continuing professional development (CME) – take relevant courses

3. Self-directed learning groups

4. Appraisal/revalidation

5. Experience – continuing process

6. Sitting the MRCGP exam. Fellowship by assessment.

What is a personal development plan?

- Identification of a learning need.
- Determine how I have established this need.
- Set specific aims/learning objectives.
- Determine how I will achieve these objectives.
- It is based on learning cycles of which we have ownership.
- Evaluate out learning cycle/development plan.
- Determine the time scale.
- It is part of revalidation.

Realistic objectives are achievable if you follow the acronym: SMART:

- Specific – clear and concise
- Measurable
- Achievable – check resources
- Realistic
- Time-related – set dates

What is the evidence that we are good at self-appraisal?

We are clearly not good at self-appraisal. Tracy et al in Australia showed that the majority of doctors who stated that they were good at endoscopies got the multiple choice questions (MCQs) wrong. Quote articles to gain merit points!

- (Pt unmet needs) (Doctor Educat needs).
- PUNS & DENS diaely
- Attend Courses
        objective exams - MRCGP.
- Do Audits.
  There are several ways I keep uptodate.

17. A 60-year-old woman is noted to have a breast lump on exam, which is highly suspicious in nature. You would like her to attend hospital but she is adamant she only wants homeopathy. Discuss the issues. (Professional values/care of patients)

The implications for me as the doctor are my feelings and my desire to do no harm. I acknowledge this patient would make me feel angry. I do not know enough about homeopathy to understand its benefits/complications.

The implications for the patient are the patient's health and embarking on a treatment which is not proven to be effective in breast cancer. I acknowledge the specific ethical issues:

1. **Autonomy** – I acknowledge that the patient has a right to choose.

2. **Beneficence** – But I would still wish to do good and would try to persuade her to allow me to refer her to the breast clinic also.

3. **Consent/competence** – I would obtain her consent to refer her to the hospital. I would ensure that she was making a competent decision.

4. **Do no harm** – I would need to ensure that homeopathy would not be deleterious to the patient, i.e. poison her.

5. **Equity** – ensure equal access to all if I refer one patient to homeopathy.

Cost implications for the practice

I would discuss this patient with my colleagues (partners) and consult the MDU as regards the medicolegal implications. I would ask her to return after I had obtained sufficient information from my partners, the MDU and written information on homeopathy. When she returns, I would try to negotiate and reach a compromise – perhaps refer her both to homeopathy and to the breast clinic.

Implications for the practice

These are the costs of homeopathy and other alternative treatments.

Implications for society

The cost.

What is a patient's perception of health influenced by? (Society/communication)

The past, family, hospital, Internet, media, press and often results in a consumer's perception.

Pts' have right to request but Doctor
helps pts to make informed decisions.

Samuel Hahnemann → Came auto homeopathy.
In Aug 27 2005 in Lancet proven
→ that homeopathy effect is = to
placebo effect.

18. What is the difference between a patient and a consumer?

Simply put, the difference between a patient and a consumer is that the patient comes with 'needs' for advice, health intervention etc., but the consumer has 'wants', often financially motivated. Consumers expect 24/7 service, and want to set the agenda. The consumer is always 'right', which means that if consultations were led in this manner, the agenda would be entirely patient centred. This would lead to the detriment of the session with consultations over-running, unreal expectations asked of the doctor and burnout for GPs. Consumers are responsible only to themselves and to society. Patients, on the other hand, also want direct access and less waiting time but are prepared to negotiate and wait. They are responsible to the health service, as their needs impact on the availability of services for others. You could mention the theory of right vs the theory of utility. Patients should be allowed to participate in the shaping of the health service and better understand the difficult role of gate keeping/ rationing for the individual GP.

19. How do patients put doctors at risk? (Personal responsibility/ communication)

1. **Mental** – stress, burnout, verbal abuse, threats, litigation.
2. **Physical** – violence, human immunodeficiency virus (HIV), hepatitis, viruses, severe acute respiratory syndrome (SARS).

What are your strategies to manage a violent patient?

I would hope that the situation would not escalate to the point that a patient becomes violent. I would position myself sideways to the patient to appear less aggressive. I would soften and lower my tone of voice. I would breathe in and out slowly to appear calm and self-controlled. I would appear to be listening to the patient by nodding, tilting my head sideways, wrinkling my forehead, and squinting. I would make myself aware of the signs that the patient is about to use force (marching to and fro, scuffling his feet, punching his fists, flushed face, negative chanting (saying 'You people don't care,' repeated over and over in an attempt to dehumanise me). If this occurs, I would press the alarm button and try to exit the room. If he approaches me menacingly, I would exhale, inhale and then shout 'Back!' and hopefully take him by surprise, so that I could flee.

What would you do before you see your next patient?

I would make a record of the encounter in writing in the incident book for future critical event analysis to be discussed at the next practice meeting. In my surgery we have a zero tolerance to violence. The patient would face instant removal from the list. I would talk to another partner (debrief). I would use Neighbour's technique of housekeeping. I would have a time out and walk around the surgery or drink a cup of coffee and make sure I was mentally prepared to see the next patient.

20. What is wrong with doctors doing drugs? (Care of patients, personal responsibility/ professional values)

Implications for the doctor

This impairs clinical judgement, possibility of being struck off by the GMC, endangers his health, family discord, etc.

Implications for the patient

It endangers the health and life of his patients, and results in poor patient satisfaction and poor clinical care of patients.

Implications for the practice

An increase in litigation and unwelcome press coverage.

Implications for society

There is a medicolegal responsibility to report the doctor to the GMC and for the doctor to take personal responsibility for his health and contact the GMC.

21. How do you feel about quality pay for good GPs? (Professional values/society)

I am in support of this form of positive reinforcement.

What are some quality markers?

- Access to building/handicapped access
- APD
- Appointment availability – 48-hour access (but is it really better to see a locum than your own GP? Is this really a good quality measure?)
- Disease registers for coronary heart disease (CHD), diabetes, etc.
- Length of consultations
- PACT – prescribing patterns (not a good indicator in different populations; what if a more expensive drug is better?) Prescribing data does not follow a Gaussian curve; this is because it is a proxy measure and not a direct measure of quality data. Some drugs cost more than others. So to determine how far your practice is away from the mean can only be a relative measure and does not reflect a true accurate account of prescribing.
- Patient surveys of practice/GP
- Reaching screening targets
- Referral patterns (a GP with specialist dermatology interest may make more referrals to a dermatology clinic because he has more knowledge of the services available in the hospital in that particular area. Does this make him a worse GP?)
- Waiting lists

How else can you assess GPs?

- Accredited Professional Development – an initiative developed by the Royal College of General Practitioners (RCGP)
- Clinical Governance
- Fellowship by Assessment
- Membership by Assessment of Performance
- Quality Practice Award
- Quality Team Award

22. The nurse complains to you that the nurse practitioner always leaves the treatment room dirty. How would you handle the matter? (Communication/working with colleagues)

I would follow my practice-based in-house complaints procedure. I would ask her to put the complaint in writing to the practice manager with a copy for the nurse practitioner as soon as possible. I will inform her that the complaint will be logged. The practice manager will then discuss the complaint with the partners and would ask the nurse practitioner to respond in writing. The manager will investigate the complaint. The matter should be addressed within 10 working days or else the manager will explain to the nurse the reason for the delay and will indicate how much longer is needed.

I would hope that the nurse practitioner would meet with the nurse, apologise and make necessary changes to her practice. If the issue is not resolved in this matter, then I would arrange a practice meeting to address all members of the health team with regards to the practice policy on health and safety standards for the practice and issue a written warning to the nurse practitioner after mutual agreement with the partners and practice manager.

23. Would you accept a gift from a patient? (Professional value/ personal responsibility)

Do not get into an auction with the examiner! The examiner may rattle off a list of gifts and ask you what you would and would not be prepared to accept. If you get into this monetary auction, you are going in circles and missing the point. Do not get rattled! The correct answer is that it is a subjective decision. Yes, I would accept, if I felt comfortable that the nature of the gift was in proportion with the services I had provided and did not make me feel uneasy. But it would also depend on the attitudes of the patient, practice and society. I would initially question whether the patient had any hidden agenda (past and present knowledge of patient's consultations), whether this gift was a bribe (size of the gift) and whether this patient was crossing the boundary? If I were led to suspect this, I would inform the patient that according to the General Medical Services contract, the patient is entitled to free care, and that I could not accept a gift if the patient expected preferential treatment. If the gift was given for Christmas, or following help given with a family bereavement, this would be acceptable.

Giving gifts depends on the culture and age of the patient. Elderly people are more inclined to giving gifts as they recall when there was no NHS and medicine was private. I would try not to offend a patient by refusing an appropriate gift and would add that I would be putting the cash in the practice kitty or sharing the bottle of wine with the practice. I would follow the practice agreement on acceptance of gifts. I am aware that according to the Health and Social Care Bill 2001, all gifts > £100 in value should be registered and gifts > £25 should be declared.

ABPI Industry makes it illegal for drug reps to give gift > 6£ & > 3 times/ a year.

Emotional intelligence by Daniel Goldman

Blink by Malcolm Gladwell
About Psychology

24. What is appraisal? Revalidation? (Personal and professional growth/care of patients, working with colleagues)

Appraisal

This is an annual 'positive process to give GPs feedback on their past performance, to chart their continuing progress and to identify development needs.'

Appraisal forms for GPs working for the NHS may be downloaded off www.doh.gov.uk/appraisal. Appraisal covers the seven areas of good medical practice under the headings of good clinical care, maintaining good medical practice, relationships with patients, working with colleagues, teaching and training, probity, and health. This 23-page document is then sent to a GP appraisor (list from PCT), who will then arrange a meeting with the GP appraisee. At the end of the document is the personal development plan; suggest to list two items. The summary form is then sent to the supervisor of the appraisor.

Revalidation

This is a 5-yearly process and if you have had five annual appraisals, this process should be straightforward. This tests 'fitness to practice.' Few will fail. You will fail if you pose a danger and risk to patients if allowed to continue to practice. On average this amounts to 1–2 doctors per PCT. Revalidation uses materials from appraisals so keep all evidence of audits, educational activities, evidence of development, etc. in one place.

Online MCQ paper
Audits
Pt satisfaction survey

} few tools for
revalidation.

25. Would you whistle-blow on an alcoholic partner? (Working with colleagues/personal responsibility)

Why now?

Verify the suspicion with evidence: patients/colleagues reports/complaints poor clinical judgement, mistakes.

How?

It affects the doctor, partners, patients and practice. Does the doctor have insight? Arrange a partner meeting.

Who to approach?

Approach the Medicolegal Advisory Service for advice, the Dean for a poorly performing doctor, the local PCT advisor, and the GMC. You are protected by the Whistleblowing Act and you owe a duty of care to patients if you know a colleague is unwell.

What to do?

Contact the PCT, MDU and GMC. Notify the doctor in question of your actions and suggest he call the BMA counseling services, National Clinical Assessment Authority (NCAA), national counseling service for sick doctors, sick doctors trust, doctors support network, etc.

The GMC will arrange for a medical screener to appoint two GMC examiners (the doctor in question may also appoint if he or she wishes) to investigate the matter and decide on the doctor's fitness to practice. The examiners may then recommend that a medical supervisor be assigned to the doctor. If the supervisor finds that the doctor's ability to practice continues to deteriorate or the doctor refuses to have a supervisor, a health committee of seven medical personnel and two laypeople will meet to discuss the case.

26. A 10-year-old girl is dying of leukaemia. Her mother asks you for your home telephone number so she can call you if things get worse. Would you give it to her? (Professional values/personal responsibility)

Patient issues

I would want to know why she wants my number. Is she dependent on you? Is she more comfortable calling you than the emergency services? Why can't she cope? Her response is that she just wants to talk to you in case she dies.

Society/medicolegal issues

I have to consider the medicolegal issues if she calls and I am not at home. Do I also give her my mobile number? If I give her my phone number, I am setting a precedence and she may call me instead of attending the surgery. The worst scenario is that I underestimate a 'tummy ache' over the phone and she does not attend surgery and instead dies of a perforated ulcer! I have to consider equity to all patients, so this precedence would allow other patients access to my home number and mobile.

Triage bypass Caed

Personal/doctor issues

I also have to consider my health and being 'on call' for this particular patient during unsociable hours, and the potential risk of burnout if my family and personal life is interrupted repeatedly.

In conclusion, my answer is that I would not give out my home number to the mother but inform her that the surgery can get hold of me if I am on call or in the surgery, or take a message if I am not available, so that I can return her call. If I am particularly close to the family, I would give my mobile number to the out-of-hours co-op, so that if the daughter passes away after hours, I may be contacted and attend the family in person to offer my support.

Can give mobile no to out of hrs service only for bereavement services.

27. A 14-year-old girl asks you for contraception. What would you do? (Communication/care of patients)

Competence

A guidance report entitled *Confidentiality and People Under 16* issued jointly by the BMA, GMSC, Health Education Authority (HEA), Brook Advisory Centres, FPA and Royal College of GPs (RCGP) gives a step-by-step approach to this important ethical issue. I need to assess her for Frazer competence to consent to treatment. Competence is determined in terms of the patient's ability to understand the choices and their consequences, including the nature, purpose and possible risks of any treatment (or non-treatment). The legal position dictates that I need to determine whether she understands the potential risks and benefits of the treatment and the advice given.

Confidentiality

I need to stress at all times the value of parental support and explore reasons why the patient is unwilling. I will advise her that I am respecting her confidentiality.

Unprotected sexual intercourse

I need to take into account whether she is likely to have sexual intercourse without contraception, and whether her physical or mental health, or both, are likely to suffer if she does not receive contraceptive advice or supplies. I must also consider whether the patient's best interests would require the provision of contraceptive advice or methods or both without parental consent.

Ideas, concerns and expectations

I would explore her ideas, concerns and expectations with contraception. I would consider whether there was a hidden agenda?

Under-age sex +/– consent, abuse?

I would ask for the age of her male partner as I am legally bound to report any underage sex with an older man with the advice of the MDU.

If pt < 13 having sex inform Police immediately .
17y partner Explain, provide guidance. 18y → Child Prot

Duty of care if there is a question of abuse

I would inform the Child Protection Agency.

Emergency contraception

I would determine whether she is really asking for emergency contraception or regular contraception. If she is here for emergency contraception, I would determine whether unprotected sexual intercourse (UPSI) has occurred within 3 days for Levonelle-2 or within 5 days for the coil and check her blood pressure (BP) and weight before prescribing emergency contraception (EC) (one tablet to be taken immediately and the second tablet in 12 hours).

Pregnancy

I would perform a urine pregnancy test if she has missed a period or to exclude pregnancy prior to prescribing regular contraception.

Contraception/sexually transmitted diseases

If she is here for regular contraception, I would describe to her the various options in contraception and give her pamphlets to read. In surgery, I would take a full history to assess for contraindications, check her BP and weight, check a urine pregnancy test (UPT) and advise her to commence regular contraception on day 1 of her next period. I would give advice on missed pills, concurrent antibiotics, diarrhoea or vomiting and cover potential side effects.

I would repeatedly encourage her to inform her parents, but would reassure her that the consultation is confidential, and I will not be informing her parents. I would also advise her to always have her male partner use condoms to protect herself from STDs.

28. What qualities are needed to be a good leader? (Communication/working with colleagues)

1. **Blake and Maslow's Humanistic Theory** – direct and motivate, increase one's sense of personal worth, use of rewards, set goals.

2. **Burns and Tichy's Psychoanalytic Theory** – the transformational leader transcends his own interests for the good of the group, to identify the good qualities/abilities in one's colleagues and incorporate these with a plan.

3. List of leadership traits:

   - Ability to conduct effective meetings
   - Ability to deal with conflict positively
   - Ability to inspire trust
   - Ability to tolerate uncertainty
   - Acceptance of responsibility
   - Assertiveness
   - Calmness under pressure
   - Capability
   - Ability to coax
   - Ability to compare
   - Ability to concentrate
   - Ability to control
   - Dependability
   - An enthusiastic motivator
   - An excellent communicator and listener
   - Flexibility
   - Good organisational skills
   - Good sense of humour
   - Knowledgeable
   - Self-confidence
   - Sociability

29. What are the different types of team members? How do you manage conflict within a team? (Communication/working with colleagues)

Belbin (1981) describes eight types of team members:

1. Completer–finisher (conscientious, orderly)

2. Co-ordinator (calm, self-confident team-controller)

3. Implementer (dutiful organiser)

4. Monitor–evaluator (unemotional problem analyser)

5. Plant (unorthodox problem-solver)

6. Resource investigator

7. Shaper (dynamic, slave-driver)

8. Teamworker (sensitive, internal facilitator).

Bransford and Stein (1984) suggested the IDEAL model for managing conflict/solving problems:

1. Identify the problem.

2. Define the problem.

3. Explore possible strategies.

4. Act on the strategies.

5. Look back and evaluate the effects.

Other strategies for managing conflict include accommodation, avoidance, collaboration, competition, and compromise. However the best solution is a win-win solution and not a compromise, and to do this one has to ask the question, 'why?': 'Why is this a problem?' 'Why can't you change?' 'Why is this upsetting you?'

30. What is the role of the GP in rationing? (Professional values/ society)

The GP plays a vital role in the rationing or limiting of healthcare resources to society. One means is by prescribing generically. I am aware that I wear two hats – clearly one on behalf of the patient sitting in front of me and one to ensure equity to the wider society. I am aware that sometimes I will make that extra effort on behalf of one patient to get that person seen sooner by the hospital and factors that influence me in making that decision are gravity of illness, risk of malignancy, severity of pain, and frequency of GP visits. But I am also aware that I have a personal responsibility to manage my financial portion of the healthcare budget. I can sometimes resort to hiding behind PCT guidelines when faced with a difficult decision.

Barbara Starfield research showed that systems that give right of referral to GPs with gatekeeper function are more efficient in use of the nation's wealth for healthcare, lower healthcare costs and better healthcare outcomes.

31. You come across a cervical smear result of severe dyskaryosis that has been filed away without being addressed. What do you do with this information? (Professional values/care of patient)

I would take personal responsibility for this incident and call the patient to come in to discuss this matter. Non-disclosure is only justified if it is felt that the information would be likely to cause serious harm to mental health. In this case, I would disclose the mistake to her. I would explain to her that an oversight had occurred and explain the implications of a smear result with severe dyskaryosis. I would apologise to her for this mistake. I would then fax an urgent referral form for colposcopy and would try to obtain an appointment for her by phone, while she is in my surgery.

I would explain that the practice would have a critical incident review meeting to both review and change their current policy for receiving and reviewing smear results, to ensure this mistake cannot happen again. After the consultation, I would complete a critical incident form and bring up this matter at the next practice meeting, ensuring that all relevant staff are in attendance. A new protocol with a safety-net would then be devised, implemented and reviewed. For example, a logbook should be kept of all patients who have smear tests. Results should be reviewed by both the practice nurse and GP, and the results and action to be taken should be logged in this book and reviewed weekly by a designated person. It will then be clear if results have not been received or if an action has not occurred.

I would take ownership of the result.
offer minutes of meeting of SEA to pt.
offer her that she can lodge an official
complaint.
in the end.

32. How do you keep to time? (Personal responsibility, care of patients)

- I would have a clock in front of me either on the computer screen or on a shelf, so that I make myself aware of the time.

- I would manage patients with long lists, by asking them to list their problems first. I would assess and prioritise their list. I would then remind them that they have booked a 10-minute appointment and for them to select the most important one or two items on their list. Hopefully this will coincide with my assessment of which matters need tending to the most and which may be dealt with at a later consultation.

- I would allow the patients to have their say for at least 90 seconds and then give direction to the consultation.

- If patients are more than 10 minutes late, I would ask the receptionist to re-book them or place them on the emergency list if the matter is life-threatening.

- I would reserve some flexibility in time management, depending on the nature of the condition with which the patient presents, as I know that some problems may require more than 10 minutes and hope to make up this time with shorter consultations later in that session.

- I dictate my referral letters with the patient in the room, as the problem is still fresh in my head. The patient can correct any errors in address, phone number or information I am dictating. It saves on admin time later.

- In between patients, I like to use Neighbour's strategy of housekeeping. I clear my mind, get up and walk around the room, make phone calls or take a tea or loo break. I find that I am in a better and more efficient state of mind when seeing the next patient. Poor time management can lead to stress and burnout, and should be avoided.

33. What do you know about clinical governance? Commission for Health Improvement? National Institute of Clinical Excellence? PACT? NHS plan? (Society, personal and professional growth)

Definitions

Clinical governance is the initiative of the White Paper, *The New NHS: Modern and Dependable*. It is a framework to improve patient care through high standards. It promotes personal and team development, cost-effective, evidence-based clinical practice, risk avoidance and the investigation of adverse situations.

The **Commission for Health Improvement** (CHI) oversees the quality of clinical governance and of services. It reviews all types of organisations including the PCT, hospitals and GP practices for quality of services to patients.

GPC (GMSC) – is the General Practitioners' Committee and is the sole negotiating body between GPs and the Department of Health. It is a standing body of the BMA and represents all GPs.

LMC – the Local Medical Committee is a statutory body of locally elected GPs who meet monthly and annually at a national conference.

NHS Plan (2000–2010)

1. **Patient's perspective** – 3000 modern practices, decreased waiting lists, NICE, SMART cards, Patient Advocacy and Liaison Services (PALS), 7000 extra beds, 100 new hospitals, NHS Direct, out-of-hours pharmacies, review of complaints procedures.

2. **Professionals** – GP access < 48 hours, specialist GPs, information technology (IT) electronic booking and links to hospitals, increased personal medical services (PMS) (now the new GP contract), abolish single-handed GPs, National Service Framework (NSF) targets, PCTs care trusts, nurse practitioners, 2000 more GPs.

3. **Performance** – clinical governance (audit, annual appraisals), NCAA to assess doctors' performance quickly to avoid years of suspension during an enquiry, protocols, green–yellow–red practices.

4. **Prevention** – NSF for mental health, coronary heart disease, old age, cancer etc., better distribution of GPs to deprived areas, Golden Handshake incentive, priority given to alcohol/drug strategies, teenage pregnancy, HIV and to stop smoking.

NICE produces and disseminates clinical guidelines to promote cost-effective therapies and uniform clinical standards. It gives guidance on health technologies, clinical management of specific conditions, and referrals from primary to secondary care.

PACT, prescribing analysis and cost data of prescribing patterns, is a document issued to each GP practice which gives a summary of the practice's prescribing patterns. It highlights percentage of generic vs brand-name prescribing, annual expenditures, categories types of prescriptions and compares the practice prescribing patterns to those of local practices in the PCT.

34. What is the role of the community pharmacist? (Professional values/working with colleagues)

- Community pharmacists have access to healthy people and therefore can be used to promote health.
- First port of call for patients.
- Educate patients regarding medication.
- Facilitate responsible self-medication.
- Monitor dosage. Can be used as a safety-net if doctors prescribe the incorrect dose.
- Collect and deliver home prescriptions.
- Decrease frequency of GP consultations by managing minor ailments.
- Stop prescription wastage (cost-effective prescribing).
- Relay information regarding patient's views on returned drugs to the pharmacy.
- May issue emergency contraception.

also offer H. Pylori test

CO testing on people on NRT

Check INR
medication reviews
Can issue Statins.
In Manchester Viagra

35. A patient's mother demands antibiotics for the child's sore throat. What skills can you use? (Care of patient/ communication)

- Non-verbal communication – body language, listen to patient's mother's perception of antibiotics, nod, use good eye contact, focussed attention, smile, etc. Use non-threatening body language and appear to listen with a furrowed brow, tilted head, etc., to diffuse a potentially angry patient.

- Verbal communication – echoing, reflect, summarise, and use SCORES.

- Use consultation models, i.e. Bower and Bower (DESC – describe, explain why you are concerned, specify one change, consequences).

- Use clinical skills to demonstrate whether antibiotics are necessary or not. Explain taking into account the patient's mother's understanding of health and antibiotics.

- Conflict management (accommodate, avoid, collaborate, compete, compromise, etc.).

- Advise mother of options besides antibiotics. Share management options.

- Gift-wrapping – say 'Your daughter has avoided those "nasty" antibiotics this time.'

- Recognise when the consultation has been a success.

36. What are the pros and cons of using e-mail in day-to-day practice? (Communication/care of patients/working with colleagues)

Pros

- Quick, formal form of communication within the practice
- Avoids losing bits of paper
- Minimises interruption/distraction
- Patient can directly communicate with the doctor during and out-of-hours (OOHs)
- Doctors can communicate with each other (hospital and GP) for advice
- NHS Intranet/GP links to electronic booking expedite appointments
- Cost-effectiveness
- Paperless

Cons

- Problem with confidentiality
- Who has right of access?
- Not all patients have access to computers.
- Cannot tell from an e-mail the level of a patient's distress as one can from a phone call.
- Computers can crash – loss of data. A huge memory space is needed to store necessary information.
- Cost issue of equipment.
- Doctors need to acknowledge every e-mail from patients, partners, hospital. Is this making more work?

37. What makes for a successful practice meeting? (Communication/working with colleagues)

- Previous experience
- Plan ahead
- Pre-notification/ pre-meeting to set agenda and give notice
- Preparation – realistic agenda, prioritise agenda, no distractions, all voices heard equally, time management
- Processing – good leader, ownership, dynamics of group
- Putting it on record – decisions made, taking minutes, delegate responsibility of tasks.

38. A patient presents to you depressed and with suidical ideation. He admits that he has had an affair with his 15-year-old pupil. What will you do? (Professional values, care of patients)

Issues for the patient

- Why is he disclosing this now?
- Confidentiality
- Is the pupil registered at the practice?
- Sexually transmitted disease (STDs)
- Mental state exam

Issues for the doctor

- Neighbour's model of housekeeping 'What baggage do I bring?'
- My personal views should not cloud my judgement.
- Giving non-judgemental care.
- Doctor–patient relationship.
- Discuss with partners.
- Legally bound to report under-age sex.
- Acknowledge feelings of disgust.

Issues for the practice/society

The patient is a paedophile. The Children's Act ensures safety of children.

Legal issues

- It is the GP's duty to breach confidentiality and discuss the case with the police.
- Discuss the matter with the MDU.

Ethical issues

- Autonomy (premorbid state of the patient, mental state)
- Beneficence (help patient in the long term)
- Consent (was the pupil consenting to sex?)
- Duty of confidentiality (breach)
- Equity (justice, legal obligation to protect child).

Plan

- Inform the patient.
- Admit the patient to a psychiatric hospital under section 2 and notify a section 12 doctor.
- Get a psychiatrist to assess the patient's mental state.
- Ring the MDU before you call the police.
- Notify the police. but do not tell pt.

Contact crisis team.

Info   find out about 15 yr old if she is
                        our pt → child protection
                                        services
If other agency → inform the agency.

39. What is an audit? (Personal and professional growth/care of patients)

Audit can be used as a quality tool in healthcare. It looks at the structure, process and outcome. Specifically, audit criteria includes:

- Identification of the problem
- Selection of the topics
- Literature review
- Definition of criteria
- Set/reset standards
- Collection of data
- Comparing results to standards
- Planning changes to organisation
- Close the loop by going back to the set/reset standards step.

40. You discover that a community nurse is misusing controlled drugs. What do you do? (Professional values/working with colleagues)

This question asks you if you would whistle-blow on a colleague:

- Assess hard evidence. Corroborate
- Discuss with all the partners.
- Contact the BMA with regard to employment issues.
- Contact the Royal College of Nursing.
- Contact the MDU.
- Contact the PCT.
- Discuss this matter with the nurse and the need for you to report this. If she is under your employment, you may suspend her. If the community nurse is employed by the PCT, contact the BMA first for advice.

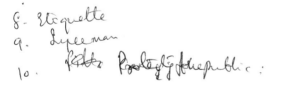

1st inform PCT to suspend the nurse.
        whistleblow to NMC.

8 - Etiquette
9 - Dipeeman
10 · Protect Protecting the public.

41. What are the communication methods available in your practice? (Communication/ working with colleagues)

- Appraisals
- Complaints procedures
- Computer – e-mail, instant messages
- Face-to-face (verbal)
- Message books
- Practice meeting with minutes distributed or posted
- Significant events analysis
- Telephone
- Written memos

The decision to choose one method over the other depends on both the timing or urgency of the matter to be addressed and the sensitivity of the content. I would classify matters as urgent, soon or routine. I would also determine which items need to be communicated to one person in particular vs the entire practice.

A formal practice meeting would be more appropriate to discuss changes to the practice, such as a new walk-in clinic for teenagers, etc. There should be equal agreement (equity) among practice staff when to use which method of communication. Failure to communicate can result in mistakes and having a good, organised practice with a protocol for effective information transfer will minimise this risk.

42. A 40-year-old daughter requests opiates for her mother, who has sustained a suspected fractured pelvis and does not want hospital care. The mother is demented. What would you do? (Professional values/care of patients)

This is yet another ethical question. Don't forget to quote theories for extra points. The most popular ethical framework to quote is that of two American ethicists, Beauchamp and Childress. Their four principles are:

1. **Autonomy** (allow people to determine their own futures) – confidentiality, decision sharing, informed consent.

2. **Beneficence** (do good) – cure, palliate, comfort, show compassion, show empathy, treat patients with dignity.

3. **Justice** (act fairly) – ethical rationing, fairness, treat equals equally, treat non-equals unequally in proportion to the degree of inequality.

4. **Non-maleficence** (do no harm) – non-harm, non-iatrogenesis.

The four moral theories are:

1. **Theory of duties/deontology** – this describes rules of moral conduct as codified in the GMC regulations. It states that the important thing ethically is not consequences but our willingness to follow rules or honour duties. My responsibility is to keep to the rules. This gives rise to conflict between deontology and consequentialism in such cases as euthanasia and surrogacy.

2. **Theory of rights** – this describes the social rights of people to receive certain services.

3. **Theory of utility/consequentialism** – this describes what is morally good in terms of the greatest good for the greatest number. Utilitarianism, a variant theory, states that the good consequence to maximise is the amount of happiness for the individuals involved.

4. **Theory of virtue** – this describes innate GP characteristics such as caritas.

In any ethical decision-making process, follow the steps listed below:

- Is this an ethical question?

- Who are all the people involved?
- What are all possible solutions?
- Assess the pros and cons to each solution using the four principles of Beauchamp and Childress.
- Make a decision using the consequentialist or deontology theory.
- Discuss your decision with colleagues.
- Check the precedents with the GMC, MDU, BMA, etc.
- Make a final decision.
- Impart the information to the patient in an ethical manner.
- Record everything.

In this particular case, discuss the issues for:

1. **Patient** – does she have advance directives? Assess her quality of life. Does she have carers or other support in place? How ill is she clinically?

2. **Daughter** – Does she have a hidden agenda? Is she a carer who is not coping? How does the stress of being a carer affect her own children? Does she have power of attorney? Does she have a fear of hospitals? Is she harbouring feelings of guilt? What is the family's cultural background?

3. **Practice/wider issues** – practice guidelines. Call the BMA and MDU. Consider assessment of the patient by the Care of the Elderly team. Talk to a geriatric consultant. Document everything.

43. What is a patient-centred consultation? (Communication/ care of patients)

A patient-centred consultation is one in which the patient comes with an average of five problems and represents a consultation which encompasses the patient's health beliefs.

Why do patients present?

They present at the limit of their anxiety, the limit of their tolerance to the condition or to pain, as a ticket of admission or for administrative reasons.

What is the doctor's agenda?

The doctor has both his private agenda and that of the patient's database. His private agenda includes external pressures, practice considerations, paternalism, a personal agenda (tired), and health promotion. The patient's database includes the present complaint, risk factors, and continuing and dormant problems.

What do you know about the patient's learning cycle?

They start with a change in health understanding, i.e. 'There is something wrong with me.' They then seek to address this with alternative therapies, self-care or decide to see the doctor with their ideas, concerns, and expectations. The doctor and patient should then negotiate in the consultation to make intermediate and long-term changes.

What is your favourite consultation model and how do you incorporate it into your practice?

See page 12. I like Neighbour's The Inner Consultation and incorporate safety-netting into my practice when dealing with uncertainty. I always have a back-up plan and inform the patient what to do if x, y, or z occurs.

44. Are patient participation groups a good idea? (Communication/society)

- Yes, they allow patients and people in the community to give both positive and negative feedback to the practice.
- They allow health professionals to assess the needs of the community.
- They allow practices to improve services and highlight gaps in services.
- A large enough group can lobby for changes on a wider scale and with the local MP.
- The disadvantage is the difficulty to know that the selected group is an appropriate representation of the local community. Children and the elderly may find it difficult to be heard.

+ve.

(:) Can give feedback

Tudor Hart → GP from Swansea "Inverse Care people who need the law"
Care the most don't get it.
Upper middle class people come with their own private agenda.

45. (Favourite MRCGP concepts) What do we mean by futility? Ordinary and extraordinary means? Relativism? Wants and needs? (Professional values/care of patients)

Definitions

- **Futility** – If a treatment is futile due to its poor outcome, does this render it morally wrong to administer it? For instance, would you keep an elderly demented person with brain damage on a ventilator for pneumonia?

- **Ordinary and extraordinary means** – treatments may be morally dubious due to their burdensome nature. For instance would you put a central line in a demented person to administer total parenteral nutrition (TPN)?

- **Relativism** – relates to cultural and religious differences in what is wrong or right, i.e. male circumcision, euthanasia, abortion.

- **Wants and needs** – Healthcare resources are scarce and need to be allocated in a fair manner with rational non-discriminatory assessment of need.

Don't forget **double-effect**, which has been covered in an earlier question.

46. What are the different methods of learning? (Personal and professional growth/ personal responsibility)

Interactive vs passive?

- Attending courses or lectures
- Balint group
- Distance learning
- Experience
- Internet
- Multidisciplinary learning
- Patients
- Practice-based learning (audit, developing guidelines, SEA)
- Reading journals, books, etc.
- Self-directed learning groups
- Sitting in with another GP or hospital consultant (mentoring)
- Skills training
- Young principals' group
- Video analysis
- Workshops

2. MRCGP video module

Table 2 Examiner's video marking grid

PC	Tick	Performance criteria (PC)	Examples
1		Dr encourages patient's contribution	Active listening – nod, 'aha'
2	F	*Dr responds to cues (MERIT)*	'Oh, problems at work?' 'Is there anything else?' No cues in follow-up consultation so use new pts.
3		Dr elicits appropriate details to place complaint in social and psychological context	'Is it affecting work, day to day, social life?' There are no psychosocial issues to explore with a low challenge problem, i.e. spot on a finger
4	F	Dr explores patient's health understanding	'What are you worried about?' 'What do you think is going on?' 'What do you expect from me today?' Explore ICE (patient's ideas, concerns, expectations)
5		Dr obtains sufficient information for no serious conditions to be missed	Case selection. Demonstrate a consultation which could be serious, meaty. No spot on toe, med certs, or simple rash. If the patient reports HA, ask about vomiting
6		Dr chooses an appropriate physical and mental examination	Mental state exam counts as an exam. Everyone gets tick here
7		Dr makes clinically appropriate working diagnosis	i.e. stress-related headache It doesn't have to be a flash diagnosis. If you get the diagnosis wrong, you just get no tick here
8		Dr explains diagnosis in appropriate language	Management and effects of treatment. Explain what is wrong: 'I think you've got angina. Do you know what that means?'
9		*Dr takes account of patient beliefs (MERIT)*	'I checked you over, and I don't think you have a brain tumour'
10		Dr seeks to confirm patient's understanding	'Does this make any sense to you?' 'What does the term diabetes mean to you?' 'What will you say to your wife when you get home?'
11		Dr uses appropriate management plan	All get a tick here
12	F	Dr involves the patient in the management plan	'The choices are we could prescribe antibiotics or wait and see. How do you feel about that?' Involve the patient with the plan, pause and invite the patient to decide
13		*Dr takes steps to enhance concordance, by exploring and responding to the patient's understanding of the treatment (MERIT)*	Not everything ends in a prescription so long as you give advice regarding OTC meds.
14		Dr specifies the conditions and interval for follow-up and review	

F = most candidates fail to obtain at least four ticks here.

The main sections of the videotaped consultation may fall under four headings – discover the reason for attendance (PC 1–4), define the clinical problem (PC 5,6), make a working diagnosis (PC 7), explain the problem (PC 8–10), address the patient's problems (PC 11,12) and effective use of the consultation (PC 13,14). The examiner's video marking grid (Table 2) demonstrates these points. Note the F's in the tick column. These are the performance criteria that most candidates fail to obtain at least four ticks out of the seven video consultations submitted, so pay closer attention to these PCs. To pass you must obtain four ticks for each of the 12 PCs. For merit you need to obtain four ticks for each of the additional three merit PCs. So mix and match your videotaped consultations to cover all PCs.

Detailed Instructions

1. Inform reception and your trainer which session(s) you would like to use for video-taping purposes.

2. Make several copies of the 'Patient Consent to Video Recording for Assessment Purposes' sheet and hand them to reception.

3. Either borrow the practice's video camcorder or use your own; digital is better for picture quality and especially if you can use the zoom lens. Place the remote control on your desk for easy access.

4. Set up the room appropriately. Do not have the computer monitor screen in direct view of the camera. Examiners have mentioned that they find the vertigo-effect of a moving computer screen very disconcerting and distracting. Try to position the screen to one side, or better yet off camera.

5. Do not film in front of a window. Your tape will come out dark with shadows and you will have to repeat your work. It has been done!

6. Make sure the camera has high-quality audio. If not, attach a portable microphone to your camcorder. The examiners are often hard of hearing.

7. Position the camera so that the patient's face is in full view of the camera and your side profile is in view. It is more important for the examiners to see the expressions on your patients' faces to assess rapport. One method is to position the camera facing the desk, with the patient's chair off to one side. Position your chair sideways turned towards the patient to avoid getting the back of you.

8. Write down the 15 PCs in bullet points with the actual questions you need to ask on a piece of paper and stick it on top of the desk or against the wall (off camera) but within easy eye contact for you.

9. **Do not** film yourself obtaining consent from the patient. This is an instant fail if you are not seen obtaining fully informed consent. Instead, prior to filming, obtain the initial consent and after the patient says bye, recall the patient for the second signature.

10. Select your cases carefully. Ensure that one case is of a child under the age of 10 (it is easier to tape a school-aged child than a crying baby) and that one case has a significant social or psychological dimension (homeless person, drug addict, depression, etc.) Avoid using patients who have poor English. Have a general idea of the kind of cases you are looking for. Older patients tend to have potentially serious conditions.

11. Time is of the essence, as you also need to conduct a surgery as well as find suitable consultations for the exam. If the patient mentions 'I'm here for a repeat prescription,' sick note, wart, mole, spot, etc., use your remote control and turn off the camera. You can then relax and expedite the consultation. Do not leave the camera rolling. You are wasting tape and adding to your homework after surgery. What you are looking for are patients who mention any of the following words: depression, abdominal pain, blood pressure, back pain, breast lump or pain, chest pain, fever symptoms, fever with rash, haemoptysis, haematemesis, headache, persistent cough, shortness of breath, weight loss. Don't waste your time filming for months on end. You will tire yourself out. Sensibly, you could find the right mix in 2 weeks! I did.

12. If you are interrupted during the consultation by phone or by a knock on the door, dismiss the tape. It is a good idea to put a sign on your door not to be interrupted as you are filming.

13. Try to memorize the 14 questions you need to ask so that they come trippingly off your tongue. Again rely on your discreetly positioned crib-sheet if you get stuck. Remember that the examiners are watching tapes for 8 hours straight in a secluded closet, so they are bound to doze off. Speak up and use the buzz words for the examiners to give you ticks for the respective PC. For example, I would declare: 'The options for treatment are: we do nothing, you try something over the counter, I prescribe you medication or I refer you. Which do you prefer?' There are always options so be inventive. You could give the patient the choice of paracetamol in capsule, soluble, syrup or tablet form.

14. If the patient starts to strip, guide the patient off camera. You do not want to spoil your video with a view of a woman's bra or a man's Y-front. Keep the camera rolling as you examine the patient off-screen. Remember that the examiners are marking what you say. So speak up behind the curtain.

15. Have a clock on your desk in front of you or keep the clock open on the monitor screen. You need to gauge 15 minutes. The examiners will only watch the first 15 minutes of your consultation. Practice makes perfect.

16. Make sure you have an end to your consultation by saying goodbye. Then use your remote to turn off the camera.

17. Submit seven videotaped sessions for the MRCGP. Those who are undertaking the single MRGCP/summative assessment route should submit a 2-hour tape with 10–12 videotaped consultations.

Remember only the first seven will be viewed by examiners for the MRCGP exam.

The next pages cover the workbook log (Table 3) and offer you detailed transcripts of actual dialogue during a videotaped consultation. Note the repetition of key questions asked by the doctor of the patient to elicit the respective PCs.

Table 3 Video assessment of consulting skills in 2004. Workbook and instructions. Example of completed workbook

Ref No.	Elapsed time	Date and clock time	Main reason for consultation and any special circumstances	Length (minutes)	Age and sex of patient	Degree of difficulty	Tick yes, if you know the patient	Tick if it was a follow-up visit
1	0 min	10/2/04 09:00	Chest infection, h/o coal workers' pneumoconiosis	15	80, M	Straightforward		
2	16 min	24/1/04 09:53	Boils, cough, depression	9	44, F	Moderate		
3	25 min	2/2/04 09:03	Left wrist sprain, snoring	10.5	52, F	Straightforward		
4	36 min	8/2/04 08:57	Cellulitis, hypertension	13.25	62, F	Moderate		
5	49 min	1/2/04 09:41	Drug-induced urticaria	7.33	49, F	Straightforward		
6	57 min	3/2/04 10:58	Child with fever and urinary tract infection symptoms, h/o vesicoureteric reflux	14.42	7, F	Moderate		
7	1h 12 min	6/1/04 09:14	Heroin drug addiction, requesting methadone and diazepam	12.66	34, M	Difficult	✓	✓
8	1h 24 min	4/2/04 10:44	Worried re: headache, dizziness, left earache, sore throat	13.5	51, F	Moderate		
9	1h 38 min	9/2/04 09:27	Worried re: breast pain, back pain, repeat Cilest ocp	10	19, F	Straightforward		
10	1h 49 min	9/2/04 10:21	Worried re: foot pain, vertigo	10	52, M	Straightforward		
11	1h 59 min	10/2/04 16:47	Worried re: bad chest Heavy smoker, prior hospitalisation	12.66	67, F	Moderate		

Consultation Summary Form

Reference number: 1

GP Registrar ID number: LDN/800/xxxxxx

Consent for video-recording the above consultation was obtained: Yes

Presenting complaint(s): Chest infection

Relevant background information: Coal worker's pneumoconioisis (No previous knowledge of patient)

Physical findings, if any: Rhonchi left base

Working diagnosis: Left basilar chest infection

Outcomes of the consultation: Antibiotic for 1 week

Health promotion: Patient to return to flu clinic with his wife for flu jab next week

Prescription: Amoxycillin 250 mg o t.d.s. × 7 days as before (same Px antibiotic as given 1 year ago; patient only weighs 8½ stone, so 500 mg dose was not issued)

In approximately 50 words, outline the setting of the consultation, what was achieved, and what issues may arise later:

The patient had a good understanding of his chest condition. I was concerned that I did not overlook the possibility of a chest tumour with his past history. His weight was stable. He had a past history of hypertension, but his BP was normal and his cholesterol was only slightly raised – 5.4. Next time I would have checked his peak flow as he was breathless.

(Summative assessment candidates) Please rate the degree of difficulty of this consultation by circling the appropriate response:

Straightforward

Consultation Summary Form

Reference number: | 2 |

GP Registrar ID number: | LDN/800/xxxxxx |

**Consent for video-recording the
above consultation was obtained:**   Yes

Presenting complaint(s):   Boils, cough

Relevant background information: Depression
On Prozac
Family history of insulin-
dependent diabetes mellitus
(IDDM)
(No previous knowledge of
patient)

Physical findings, if any: Several boils on the face
Temperature 37.5°C
Chest clear on auscultation

Working diagnosis: Boils
Flu symptoms

Outcomes of the consultation: Prescription for antibiotic

Prescription: Flucloxacillin 500 mg o q.d.s.
(#28)

**In approximately 50 words, outline the setting of the consultation, what
was achieved, and what issues may arise later:**

Her random blood glucose and cholesterol levels were normal. The cues
were stress and depression. She still had issues regarding the loss of her
mother, who died of cancer at age 69. She is also under stress (has canker
sores and boils). I should have explored these issues more but briefly
touched on the death of her mother, who survived a major operation only
to pass away. I forgot to prescribe her Zovirax cream for her canker
sores.

**(Summative assessment candidates) Please rate the degree of difficulty of
this consultation by circling the appropriate response:**

Moderate

Consultation Summary Form

Reference number: | 3 |

GP Registrar ID number: | LDN/800/xxxxxx |

Consent for video-recording the above consultation was obtained: Yes

Presenting complaint(s): Left wrist sprain
Snoring

Relevant background information: Married
No serious past medical history (PMH)
Housecleaner
(No previous knowledge of patient)

Physical findings, if any: Left wrist sprain
Redundant uvula and low-hanging posterior palate
Body mass index (BMI) 31

Working diagnosis: Left wrist sprain
Overweight and redundant uvula contributing to snoring

Outcomes of the consultation: Prescription given

Health promotion: Due for cervical smear next week
Explanation regarding snoring
Advice regarding weight loss

Prescription: ibuprofen gel 5%, apply topically q.d.s. p.r.n. (30 g)

In approximately 50 words, outline the setting of the consultation, what was achieved, and what issues may arise later:

The obvious cue or agenda was a third party, i.e. her husband. It sounded like positive 'nagging' from her husband to seek medical advice. She was reassured and had insight as to why she snores. My only criticism is that I should have checked the anatomical snuffbox, but as she pointed to her third metacarpal bone, I forgot.

(Summative assessment candidates) Please rate the degree of difficulty of this consultation by circling the appropriate response:

Straightforward

Consultation Summary Form

Reference number: | 4

GP Registrar ID number: | LDN/800/xxxxxx

Consent for video-recording the
above consultation was obtained: Yes

Presenting complaint(s): Facial rash

Relevant background information: Family history of CVA (mother
died at age 56)
Smokes 25 cigarettes/day
(No previous knowledge of
patient)

Physical findings, if any: Temperature was 38.5°C
BP 170/94
Hot, red, confluent rash over
forehead, cheeks and chin

Working diagnosis: 1. Cellulitis of the face
2. Hypertension, essential

Outcomes of the consultation: Prescription given
Blood tests taken – FBC, U/E,
LFTs, fasting lipids, ESR
Review BP in 2 weeks

Prescription: 1. Aspirin E/C 75 mg od (#28)
2. Flucloxacillin 500 mg o.d.
q.d.s. (#28)
3. Fusidic acid 2% +
hydrocortisone acetate 1%
cream topical b.d. (30 g)

In approximately 50 words, outline the setting of the consultation, what
was achieved, and what issues may arise later:

She understood that stress can bring on rashes. The cue here was that this
particular weekend had been her 40th wedding anniversary with her husband, if he were still alive. I could find no obvious cause for the infection,
although she did mention it had started in her scalp. The other cue was
that her mother had died from a CVA at the age of 56. I was surprised by
the elevated BP and decided to investigate fully and reassess her BP. I
started her on aspirin as a precaution.

(Summative assessment candidates) Please rate the degree of difficulty of
this consultation by circling the appropriate response:

Moderate

Consultation Summary Form

Reference number: | 5

GP Registrar ID number: | LDN/800/xxxxxx

Consent for video-recording the above consultation was obtained: Yes

Presenting complaint(s): General body rash and itching

Relevant background information: She had been prescribed flucloxacillin for an infected wasp sting on her leg (No previous knowledge of patient)

Physical findings, if any: Generalised rash

Working diagnosis: Drug-induced urticaria

Outcomes of the consultation: Explanation. Allergy alert on her medical records.

Prescription: 1. Piriton 4 mg o q.d.s. p.r.n. (#12)
2. Hydrocortisone 1% cream topical b.d. p.r.n. (30 g)

In approximately 50 words, outline the setting of the consultation, what was achieved, and what issues may arise later:

The cue was that she was not sure if this rash was contagious, as her daughter is pregnant. She wanted confirmation and reassurance that this was a drug reaction and how to manage it. I should have educated her as to the difference between a drug reaction and anaphylaxis, on hindsight.

(Summative assessment candidates) Please rate the degree of difficulty of this consultation by circling the appropriate response:

Straightforward

Consultation Summary Form

Reference number: | 6

GP Registrar ID number: | LDN/800/xxxxxx

**Consent for video-recording the
above consultation was obtained:**   Yes

Presenting complaint(s):   Urinary tract infection symptoms
Tiredness

Relevant background information: Vesicoureteric reflux
Normal MSU 11/03 and 12/03
(no previous knowledge of
patient)

Physical findings, if any: Temperature 37°C
Urine dipstick 1+ leu, nitr.
negative, rbc negative, ketones
negative, protein negative

Working diagnosis: Dysuria

Outcomes of the consultation: MSU was sent to the lab. I called
the next day. The result was no
organisms and no growth

Prescription: 1. Trimethoprim paediatric
suspension 50 mg/5 ml – 5 ml
nocte (100 ml)
2. Paracetamol paediatric
suspension 120 mg/5 ml – 1–2
teaspoons q.d.s. p.r.n.

**In approximately 50 words, outline the setting of the consultation, what
was achieved, and what issues may arise later:**

The cue was the child's tiredness at school, which I could have explored.
I was faced with the dilemma of treating her symptoms with a full course
of antibiotics (in view of her urological condition) or just issue her a pro-
phylactic dose, as her previous MSUs were normal. I handed over the
decision to her mother, who knew her daughter's condition and hospital
follow-up better, and reassured the mother that her daughter could have
been tired due to the fever.

**(Summative assessment candidates) Please rate the degree of difficulty of
this consultation by circling the appropriate response:**

Moderate

Consultation Summary Form

Reference number: | 7

GP Registrar ID number: | LDN/800/xxxxxx

**Consent for video-recording the
above consultation was obtained:** Yes

Presenting complaint(s): Heroin drug addiction
Requesting methadone and
diazepam

Relevant background information: Recently released from prison
Failed detox in prison
I initiated methadone therapy
after a positive urine toxicology
He has also been taking
diazepam for the past 10 years
Last urine test showed evidence
of cannabis, opiates and
methadone
(follow-up patient)

Physical findings, if any: Nil

Working diagnosis: Methadone and diazepam
detoxification

Outcomes of the consultation: Prescription issued
Urine sample taken

Health promotion: Due for second hepatitis B
vaccine in 2 weeks' time. I have
the first vaccine
Patient reviewed every fortnight
to decrease methadone and
diazepam

Prescription: 1. Blue script: Dispensed
methadone mixture 1 mg/ml at a
daily dose of 20 ml (TWENTY)
on a daily pick-up basis.
Dispense Saturday and Sunday
doses on Fridays. Total dose
280 ml (TWO HUNDRED AND
EIGHTY)

2. Printed script for diazepam 9 mg o.d. (2 weeks)

In approximately 50 words, outline the setting of the consultation, what was achieved, and what issues may arise later:

I had been in contact with his parole officer, and this patient is highly motivated to come off heroin and diazepam. He has insight and avoids his friends who use. He recognises that boredom leads him to smoke heroin. I have liaised with the local drug addiction team, as I am not an expert in this field. The patient and I came to a mutual agreement on the dosing of methadone and how slowly to wean off diazepam.

(Summative assessment candidates) Please rate the degree of difficulty of this consultation by circling the appropriate response:

Difficult

Consultation Summary Form

Reference number: 8

GP Registrar ID number: LDN/800/xxxxxx

Consent for video-recording the above consultation was obtained: Yes

Presenting complaint(s):
Dizziness
Headache without visual aura
Left earache
Sore throat

Relevant background information:
Past history of myocardial infarction (MI)
Had recently discontinued HRT
(No previous knowledge of patient)

Physical findings, if any:
BP 142/90
BMI 38.3
Left EAC occluded with wax.™
Right tympanic membrane nad.
Throat nad.
Normal neurological exam. No nystagmus.

Working diagnosis:
1. Viral illness vs rebound symptoms off HRT
2. Impacted cerumen left ear

Outcomes of the consultation:
Prescription given
Review if no better or symptoms worsen

Prescription:
1. Sodium bicarbonate otic drops apply t.d.s. p.r.n. for 1 week (10 ml)
2. Co-codamol 8/500 1–2 tabs q.d.s. p.r.n. headache

In approximately 50 words, outline the setting of the consultation, what was achieved, and what issues may arise later:

This was a 52-year-old woman who had already experienced a myocardial infarction. As the thinking behind HRT has changed now (only offer for menopausal symptoms and not for > 5 years), she was advised to discontinue – there were no proven cardiovascular benefits. I wasn't sure if her symptoms were rebound from HRT discontinuation or viral in nature. The wax in her ear might account for her dizziness and earache.

(Summative assessment candidates) Please rate the degree of difficulty of this consultation by circling the appropriate response:

Moderate

Consultation Summary Form

Reference number: | 9

GP Registrar ID number: | LDN/800/xxxxxx

Consent for video-recording the above consultation was obtained: Yes

Presenting complaint(s): Bilateral breast pain
Back pain
Repeat px Cilest

Relevant background information: (No previous knowledge of patient)

Physical findings, if any: BP 114/70
BMI 34.2
Non-smoker
Breast exam – nad, no axillary lymph nodes
Back exam – SLR 80 degrees L+R, neurological nad

Working diagnosis: Simple mechanical back pain
Mastalgia
Repeat o.c.p. prescription

Outcomes of the consultation: Advised to lose weight
Explanation and reassurance regarding mastalgia
Patient information leaflet (PILS) on back pain
Advised analgesia p.r.n.

Prescription: Repeat px for Cilest 6 × 21 o.d.
OTC evening primrose oil p.r.n. suggested

In approximately 50 words, outline the setting of the consultation, what was achieved, and what issues may arise later:

This was a 19-year-old female whose calling card was a request for repeat ocp. What struck me as odd was her unusually close relationship with her female friend. I did not pursue this. I hoped she would understand that losing weight would improve her back pain, and I reassured her with a normal breast examination for her mastalgia.

(Summative assessment candidates) Please rate the degree of difficulty of this consultation by circling the appropriate response:

Straightforward

Consultation Summary Form

Reference number: | 10 |

GP Registrar ID number: | LDN/800/xxxxxx |

**Consent for video-recording the
above consultation was obtained:** Yes

Presenting complaint(s): Foot pain
Vertigo

Relevant background information: Patient had been referred to Ear,
Nose and Throat (ENT) but had
still not received an outpatient
clinic appointment
(No previous knowledge of
patient)

Physical findings, if any: Left EAC impacted with
cerumen
Tinea pedis feet, especially
between the toes

Working diagnosis: Benign paroxysmal positional
vertigo
Tinea pedis

Outcomes of the consultation: Explanation and reassurance
Prescription issued
PILS given on athlete's foot
Suggested exercises to habituate
vertigo

Prescription: 1. Clotrimazole 1% cream to be
applied 2–3 times daily for 2–3
weeks and to continue for 14
days after fungal skin infection
has cleared (50 g)

**In approximately 50 words, outline the setting of the consultation, what
was achieved, and what issues may arise later:**

This was a 52-year-old man who did not have much understanding. I
attempted to explain how to avoid recurrent athlete's foot and tried to
reassure him that his dizziness on tilting his right ear was not serious. He
seemed anxious, as he had not heard from ENT. Next time, I will try
terbinafine cream (fungicidal). I forgot to do the Hallpike manouevre.

(Summative assessment candidates) Please rate the degree of difficulty of this consultation by circling the appropriate response:

Straightforward

Consultation Summary Form

Reference number: | 11

GP Registrar ID number: | LDN/800/xxxxxx

**Consent for video-recording the
above consultation was obtained:**   Yes

Presenting complaint(s):   'Bad chest', 'Terrible cold'

Relevant background information: Heavy smoker, 20 cigarettes/day all her life (> 40 packs/year history)
Hospitalised last year for pneumonia
H/o anaemia and hypertension
(No previous knowledge of patient)

Physical findings, if any: BP 150/78
Weight 55 kg (BMI normal)
Decreased air entry in left lung base, bilateral wheezes

Working diagnosis: URTI
Chronic bronchitis

Outcomes of the consultation: Prescription issued

Prescription: Amoxycillin 500 mg o t.d.s. (#21)

In approximately 50 words, outline the setting of the consultation, what was achieved, and what issues may arise later:

The cue was that she was relocating to Spain next month and wanted to get her chest infection cleared before then. Off camera, she told me she produces a lot of white phlegm, especially before winter. I brought up whether she had considered stopping smoking. Her understanding is that she smokes to 'calm her nerves'. These 'nerves' she describes as auditory hallucinations! If her chest does not improve on antibiotics, I would investigate further with a chest x-ray, as she is at high risk of chronic obstructive airways disease (COAD) or lung tumour.

(Summative assessment candidates) Please rate the degree of difficulty of this consultation by circling the appropriate response:

Moderate

Transcript of Consultation Reference 1

Chest infection

Doctor: How can I help you today? (PC1)

Patient (80 years old, M): It's me chest. I need antibiotics.

Doctor: I see. Is there anything else going on in your life? (PC3)

(Doctor is fishing for a cue or a hidden agenda. In most cases there will be no cue and the consultation is straightforward. Just remember that you only need four of your consultations to demonstrate an obvious cue to pass PC2.)

Patient: No, just me chest acting up doctor.

Doctor: Do you live by yourself? (PC3)

Patient: No, I have me Mrs.

Doctor: And how do you pass the time of day? (PC3)

Patient: Bit of gardening, walking.

Doctor: What did you do before you retired? (PC3)

Patient: I used to work in the coal mines. I've been to the hospital and all that. I had an x-ray, and it showed that I have black lungs. They told me I've got coal worker's lung.

Doctor: Why do you think you have a chest infection? (PC4)

Patient: Been coughing up yellow stuff, so I thought I'd better come up.

Doctor: Have you or your wife had a flu jab this year? (Health promotion)

Patient: No.

Doctor: How about you come back next week with your wife for the flu jab when you are better?

(Health promotion is not marked for the exam but it is always a nice touch to demonstrate you are a well-rounded, experienced GP.)

Patient: Alright.

Doctor: Have you lost any weight recently? (PC5)

Patient: Don't think so. I can eat and eat and don't seem to put on. Me Mrs. is a great cook.

Doctor: You do look very slim. May I weigh you today too? I'd like to keep an eye on your weight. (PC6)

Patient: No problem.

Doctor: Do you smoke? (PC5)

Patient: Packed it in a while back. Used to smoke a pack a day but can't now because of me chest.

Doctor: When was the last time you had a chest x-ray? (PC5)

Patient: Oh last year when me chest was bad. I don't have cancer or anything like that, just coal worker's lung they told me.

Doctor: Okay. Let's examine you today. May I start by taking your blood pressure?

Patient: I've had high blood pressure in the past.

(Doctor is seen using a manual sphygmomanometer to take the patient's blood pressure.)

Doctor: 130 over 80. That's fine. Could you stand up for me now please, and I'll come from behind and listen to your chest if I may. (PC6)

(Doctor auscultates patient's chest and detects left basilar rhonchi.)

Doctor: Yes, I agree with you. You do have a chest infection. Are you allergic to any antibiotics? (PC7–9)

Patient: No.

Doctor: Before I forget, can I get you to stand on the scales. I just want to keep a record of your weight. (PC6)

(Patient is seen stepping onto the set of scales.)

Doctor: 8½ stone. You are slim. That's fine. Thanks. You can have a seat now. Now the options are we wait and see if you get better on your own or we give you antibiotics. You have already stated you prefer antibiotics. Is that correct? (PC12)

Patient: Yeah. It's affecting me breathing now.

Doctor: Yes and as you say you are coughing up yellow phlegm, and I can also hear the infection in your chest. (PC10)

(Doctor prints off prescription.)

Doctor: Here is your prescription for amoxicillin. It's an antibiotic you've had before. You take it three times a day. It's easier to remember to take it with your meals. If you don't get better, what should you do?
(PC11, 13, 14)

Patient: Come back and see you.

Doctor: That's right. And on your way out don't forget to make an appointment for next week for you and your wife to get a flu jab.

Patient: Thank you doctor. Bye bye.

Transcript of Consultation Reference 2

Boils
Cough

Doctor: How can I help you today? (PC1)

Patient (44 years old, F): I have a cough I can't get rid of and now boils have appeared on my face.

Doctor: And how are things in general for you?

Patient: Oh I dunno. (Patient does not make eye contact and speaks softly in a monotonous tone. Patient sits with slumped shoulders.)

Doctor: How is your mood? You seem down? (PC2)

Patient: I get depressed. I've been on Prozac. It helps a bit.

Doctor: Is there any cause for your depression? Any stress in your life? (PC3)

Patient: My mother died recently. She had to go in for an operation and she never made it home.

Doctor: Oh dear. I'm so sorry. What happened?

Patient: They told her she had cancer. We were so happy when the operation went well, but then she got really sick and died.

Doctor: How old was she?

Patient: 69.

(Doctor seen touching the patient's arm in a sympathetic manner and pauses. In cases of bereavement, the GP's role is to be a witness to an event in the patient's life. Use silence to allow the patient to share the sadness with you. If there are matters that need to be tended to regarding an immediate death, your role is to facilitate the patient to take these actions.)

Doctor: Besides the cough and the rash on your face, is there anything else going on? (PC2)

(The doctor is pushing her luck in trying to find any other hidden agendas or cues.)

Patient: I have also got these sores in my mouth.

Doctor: Are you under stress? (PC2)

Patient: I guess you could call it that.

Doctor: What do you mean by that?

Patient: My husband and I are having problems. It's the finances.

Doctor: I see. Yes that would cause a lot of worry. May I examine you?

Patient: Yeah.

(Doctor is seen examining the face and noting a crop of boils, examining the mouth, taking a temperature and auscultating the chest.)   (PC6)

Doctor: Does diabetes run in your family?   (PC5)

Patient: Yes my father takes insulin.

Doctor: Let me check the screen. I see that you have been tested for diabetes and you are clear. Your cholesterol is also normal. That's good. Now what I've found is that yes, you quite rightly do have boils on your face, which will need treatment. I asked you about diabetes, as sometimes it might be a sign of diabetes. But you have been tested and do not have diabetes. The treatment options for the boils is an antibiotic cream or an antibiotic tablet, which is stronger. Which do you prefer?

(PC7, 8, 9, 12, 13)

Patient: Tablets please. I want to get better quickly.

Doctor: Are you allergic to any antibiotics?   (PC13)

Patient: Not that I know of.

Doctor: Fine. Now as for your cough, you do not have a fever and your chest sounds fine. I suspect you most likely have the flu. As it's a virus, take regular paracetamol and drink plenty of fluids. You also have canker sores, so I suspect the stress and depression you have been feeling has made you run down. The treatment options are to leave the canker sores alone or I can give you some acyclovir cream or a lozenge. What do you think?'   (PC7, 8, 9, 12, 13)

Patient: I'll take the cream.

Doctor: Fine.

(The doctor prints off the prescriptions.)

Doctor: Here is the prescription for flucloxacillin for the boil infection on your face. Are you on the pill?   (PC13)

(Doctor asks about the pill as she may need to advise the patient to use secondary precautions if on the combined oral contraceptive pill. Doctor is seen handing over the prescription and explaining how to take it. It is safer to use consultations that end in prescriptions to ensure you get a tick for PC14.)

Patient: No.

Doctor: Fine. Now take the antibiotic tablet four times a day for a week. Now I just want to make sure you understand what I've said as I seem to have done most of the talking. What would you tell your husband about today's visit?   (PC10)

Patient: I suppose I'd say that I have the flu, boils on my face and sores in my mouth. I'm a bit stressed and down, which could be the cause of it. The antibiotics I take for a week for my face. I guess I come back if I don't get better.

Doctor: Great. Now if you do want to see me next week to talk about your stress and depression, do feel free.

Patient: Thank you doctor. (PC14)

Doctor: Good bye.

Transcript of Consultation Reference 3

Left wrist pain
Snoring

Doctor: Hello. How can I help you this morning? (PC1)

(Opening lines have been overanalysed by GPs. In some cases, doctors are unable to 'help' the patients, so an alternative opening might be 'Why are you here?' but take care with your tone if you choose this opening. Do not use silence for the exam, as you are marked for actively eliciting the patient's reason for attendance.)

Patient (52 years old, F): Um, it's just my hand. I fell out of the bath over a week ago. It's not swollen as you can see or bruised or anything. It just hurts constantly.

Doctor: When you fell out of the bath, which way did you fall onto your hand? (PC5)

(Here I am trying to ascertain whether she fell onto an outstretched hand and may have sustained a missed Colles fracture.)

Patient: I fell out backwards. I've got a nonstick mat and slipped. I brought down the curtain and pole with me. So I think I put my hand down first, but …

Doctor: Oh no, nonstick! … yes, ahem. (Wait for her to finish.) (PC2)

Doctor: Have you taken any painkillers?

Patient: No, I don't like to.

Doctor: You don't like taking tablets. Oh so you have been suffering for a week! (PC2)

Patient: It started hurting here (points to wrist) but now it hurts here (pointing to metacarpals). I didn't go to the hospital because it was not swollen or broken. I thought it would go away.

Doctor: Oh right. If you could point with one finger where it hurts the most. What are you afraid of? (PC4)

Patient: I don't know. I was just wondering when the pain would stop.

(Examine the patient. Perform a neurovascular examination of the left hand.) (PC6)

Doctor: Put your thumb and index finger together, and I shall try to pull them apart. That's good. Now spread your fingers apart. Keep them apart and I shall try to squeeze them together. Now hold onto this slip of paper and I shall try to pull it away. Good.

Patient: Oh yeah, I got all the grips and everything. I've still been cleaning. It's just sore. You touched that sore bit. It's just that every now and then, I go pick something up and it really hurts.

Doctor: Yes.

Patient: As I say I should have gone to the hospital I suppose ...

Doctor: Does it hurt more in any particular time of the day?   (PC5)

Patient: No, no.

Doctor: And as you say it isn't swollen, but is it interfering with your work as a cleaner?   (PC3)

Patient: No, I can still do it, as I'm right handed and the majority of the work I do with my right hand. It's just that every now and again when I go to pick something up, it hurts.

Doctor: I don't think you've broken a bone. Your nerves are OK. I think it is a (PC7, 8) muscle sprain. I know you don't like taking pills. There are many options for managing your pain. You could either rest, you could use a painkiller in a gel form, which you can rub into the muscle, or you can try tablets which are stronger.   (PC11, 12, 13)

Patient: No I'd much rather have the gel.

Doctor: OK. Now, if you think the housecleaning is too much for you, you know you can sign yourself off for a week or do you need to work for financial reasons?

Patient: No, I just don't want to let people down.

Doctor: Oh, you are so considerate. They can go with a dirty house for 1 week.

(Doctor is seen to be smiling and speaking in a light-hearted manner. The patient smiles back. Using humour is a good technique to inject life into these consultations. The examiner will get the impression that you are an old hand and very experienced. It is also a good sign that the consultation is going well and that you have established rapport.)

Patient: I know but a lot of them are elderly couples.

Doctor: Oh I see. Well the gel will help. Is there anything else?   (PC2)

Patient: It just hurts. It's just annoying, and as I say I wouldn't normally come, but my partner's been moaning at me. And there is something else I wanted to ask you. I snore terribly. Is there anything that can be done? I don't snore through my nose. I snore through my mouth. (The hidden agenda now becomes apparent.)

Doctor: Has it always been a problem?

Patient: It has always been a problem. But its getting worse, because I've been getting heavier. And when I was pregnant it used to be very bad.

Doctor: So you recognise that weight does play a role in snoring, so you've been working on your weight? (PC9)

Patient: I've always been working on that but it doesn't do very much.

Doctor: Well, what I am going to do is check you for other things that cause snoring that can actually be fixed surgically. (PC6)

Patient: Such as?

Doctor: Well I shall examine you first to determine whether you have any of those problems.

Patient: I know I have large tonsils and adenoids.

Doctor: Tonsils usually are not a problem. Adults usually don't have large adenoids as they shrink during childhood, as you get older.

(Examine the patient's nasal septum and throat.)

Doctor: So one thing that can cause snoring is if the partition that separates the right and left nostril is crooked. (PC6, 8)

Doctor: Open your mouth please. Say ah. The dangling thing at the back of the mouth is long, and it can vibrate and cause you to snore. (PC8) There is an operation for it, but with an operation there are possible side effects. The operation involves cutting off the dangling thing at the back of your throat with a knife or electricity, and it is very, very painful. You need that thing to keep the back of the throat moist or you'll have a dry throat. There is also a rare complication of changing the sound of your voice. So you have to weigh the risks and the benefits. The snoring does not affect you but it does affect your partner. I do understand that.
(PC10)

Are you turning blue? Are you worried you are stopping breathing?
(PC5)

Patient: No it is the extent of the noise. It does wake him up, and it doesn't matter what position I am in. You can't just roll me over. I get it anywhere and anytime.

Doctor: There are options. If you think you would like surgery, then I can arrange a consultation with an ears, nose and throat surgeon and they can talk it through with you. (PC12)

Patient: Not after what you have told me.

Doctor: If you think, I'll try the safest thing and you try to lose a bit of weight; you could also try little measures like don't drink alcohol before bedtime. There is no magical cure. (PC12)

Patient: I have tried that spray at the back of the throat. But that didn't work. Well at least I asked.

Doctor: Yes and you can go back to your husband and tell him. Now let me get you that cream. Do you suffer from heartburn? Do you have any problems with your stomach? It's a cream, so it shouldn't be a problem. (Print off prescription.) (PC13) I notice on the screen that you are due for a pap smear. (Health promotion)

Patient: I have an appointment next week.

Doctor: Oh that's excellent. Shall we weigh you and keep an eye on your weight?

Patient: It's over 14! (standing on the scale)

Doctor: Oh just a little bit. 91 kg. And let's measure how tall you are.

Patient: I think I'm 5'4".

Doctor: Oh it's metric. Very hard to interpret for me. 167.5 cm. Now do take it easy with the wrist, because it does need to rest. It got quite a bang. You could try rest, elevation, an ice pack but it has been a week, so I think the gel should do it. Just rub it into your wrist three to four times a day as needed. It should get better by next week. And if you'd like to come back in a couple of week's time for another weigh-in, we can monitor your weight and offer dietary advice. Is that OK?   (PC13, 14)

Patient: Yes, thank you very much.

Doctor: Bye bye.

Transcript of Consultation Reference 4

Facial Rash
Hypertension

Doctor: Hello. How can I help you?   **(PC1)**

Patient (62 years old, F): Face.

Doctor: Your face. Oh my, yes. And how long has this been happening?

Patient: Friday.

Doctor: Since Friday. Okay, and has this ever happened before?

Patient: Well yes. It has but the other time it was in my head (pointing to her occiput). It seems to have gone to my face now.

Doctor: Right.

Patient: Terrible irritation in my head to start with and then it got very painful. T-gel shampoo, I kept using it and using it. Didn't stop. But now Friday it has broken out in my face. Whatever it was?

Doctor: Do you think this rash on the face has something to do with the shampoo, or what was going on previously with the scalp? What do you think is going on?   **(PC4)**

Patient: I don't know. I didn't think so because my head has not been too bad.

Doctor: What do you mean by your head. Was it itchy or flaky?

Patient: Well to start with it had been very painful but now it has eased off. Now my face looks like it has been scorched by the sun. Today the face is not as painful, but it has got more irritable.

Doctor: Could it be anything else? Have you used any products on your face?

Patient: I use Dove body wash.

Doctor: And you've used that before?

Patient: Yes. It has been a long time since I used anything new.

Doctor: Is there a rash anywhere else on your body?   **(PC5)**

Is there anything else going on in your life? Are you under a bit of stress?   **(PC2, 3)**

Patient: It's been a sad weekend. It would have been me and my husband's 40th wedding anniversary. I've been thinking a lot about him over the weekend. Nothing intentional. Just a lot of thoughts.

Doctor: Oh I'm sorry to hear that. Yes that is upsetting. Do you have family? **(PC2, 3)**

Patient: I have a daughter.

Doctor: Have you seen her over the weekend?

Patient: Yes.

Doctor: I notice on the screen that you are still smoking. Have you thought about cutting down? How many cigarettes do you smoke? (Health promotion)

Patient: About 25 cigarettes a day.

Doctor: What kind of work do you do? **(PC3)**

Patient: I am a detailer for the Department of Transport.

Doctor: Wow. Is it very busy? I can imagine it to be.

Patient: Yes, I deal with admin.

(Take temperature) **(PC6)**

Doctor: You're running a temperature of 38.5. How do you feel in yourself?

Patient: A bit rough.

Doctor: Any symptoms like body aches or pains, runny nose, cough? **(PC5)**

Patient: Nothing more except for feeling 63.

Doctor: 63 wow! You don't look it.

Doctor: I know you've got this going on in your face but can I give you an overall check-up? **(PC6)**

Patient: Yes.

Doctor: Any problems with your breathing? You're not coughing up anything? (PC5) Let's do your blood pressure. (Take blood pressure.) Does your daughter have children? How old is your daughter?

Patient: 34, 35. I keep losing count.

Doctor: Has she settled down? And she is your only child? **(PC3)**

Patient: She is.

Doctor: Besides work, what do you do for fun? **(PC3)**

Patient: Gardening, shopping and spending money.

Doctor: That's true it is the only problem with going shopping. (chuckle) (PC15) Has anyone commented on your blood pressure?

Patient: The nurse did say that it was bordering.

Doctor: It is on the high side today. Have you had any recent blood tests? **(PC5)**

Patient: I had one in April.

(Examine lungs. Ask patient to stand for examination.)

Doctor: Take a deep breath in and out. That's fine. Have your parents had any problems with their blood pressure, heart, strokes?   (PC6)

Patient: Mum had a stroke.

Doctor: How old was she?

Patient: 56. Many years ago though.

Doctor: Has anyone talked about aspirin for you?

Patient: No.

Doctor: Do you suffer from any problems with your stomach? I'd like to start you on a mini dose of aspirin to protect you from strokes. How do you feel about that?   (PC12)

Patient: Okay.

Doctor: I just need to check to see if we have any current blood test results (PC11) on you. Now for your face we have several options. We can either leave it and (PC12) see if it gets better, or we could give you some antibiotics because you are running a temperature and it does look like a bit of an infection is going on. Is it painful or sore?

Patient: It was very, very painful but now it is easing down.

Doctor: It's your choice. I can also either give you a low-dose steroid cream or calamine lotion.   (PC12)

Patient: Steroid cream please cause I have to go to work. I have been using E45 cream.

Doctor: Can you take time off work? You can sign yourself off. It is distressing to go to work like this and there is no point in putting yourself through it. You are allowed to take time off work. You can take up to a week off and then come back here if you need a further week off for a medical sick note. To sign yourself off sick, your employer can give you a self-cert sick form or you can obtain one from the social security office or you can just tell your employer.   (PC3)

Patient: That's alright.

Doctor: Let me see if you have any current blood tests on the computer. Your blood pressure hasn't been quite this high before. Your blood pressure right now is about 170 over 94. Before it was 145 over 84, so I'd like to do some blood tests to check you over. Have you ever had your cholesterol checked?   (PC5)

Patient: No.

Doctor: Have you had breakfast today?

Patient: No.

Doctor: Oh brilliant. I can check that today too. You're getting the full works. **(PC6)**

(Take blood)

Doctor: I'd like you to come back in 2 weeks to get your blood pressure rechecked. It might be because you have this infection going on or that you have a bit of stress in your life right now. **(PC14)**

Doctor: I'd like to start you on a mini dose of aspirin if that's OK? I'll send these off for you. Now let me get you those medicines. You're not allergic to penicillin? **(PC13)**

Patient: No, no.

Doctor: So you take the penicillin antibiotic tablet four times a day. The other one is the steroid cream with a touch of antibiotic in the cream. Your face will get better. Do come back in 2 weeks. I want to check your blood pressure, and I will have all the blood tests back as well. Let me quickly add that aspirin. **(PC11, 14)**

Patient: Shall I make an appointment outside?

Doctor: Yes please, for 2 weeks' time. OK so here's your aspirin prescription. It's a nice coated one for your stomach. Your stomach will like that. Take the aspirin once a day, the antibiotic four times a day for a week and apply the cream twice a day. Can you repeat that all back to me? I just want to check you have it right. **(PC10)**

Patient: I take the antibiotic for a week and use the cream twice a day. I take the aspirin every day. Thank you very much.

Transcript of Consultation Reference 5

Drug-induced urticaria

Doctor: Hello. How can I help you today? (PC1)

Patient: I have this rash all over my body and it is driving me crazy. It's so itchy.

Doctor: I see. What do you think it could be? (PC4)

Patient: Well I don't know if it had anything to do with that wasp sting on my leg. The doctor gave me something that starts with flu.

Doctor: Do you mean flucloxacillin?

Patient: Yes, that's right.

Doctor: Are you allergic to any antibiotics? (PC5)

Patient: Penicillin.

Doctor: May I look at that rash a bit more closely? (PC6)

Patient: Yes.

(Doctor is seen examining the rash and checks for blanching.)

Doctor: Yes, I think you're right about the cause of the rash. You're allergic to penicillin, and flucloxacillin is in the same class as penicillin! Does that make sense?

Patient: Oh! (PC9)

(Patient's facial expression shows she understands the connection.)

Doctor: Yes, so it seems as though you have an allergic rash. I'll make a quick note of your allergy on your computer records, before I forget. (PC7, 8)

(Doctor adds a drug allergy alert to the patient's medical records.)

Doctor: What was your concern regarding the rash? (PC2)

(Doctor is fishing for a cue, a hidden agenda.)

Patient: Well, I wasn't sure whether the rash was contagious. You see my daughter is pregnant, and I don't want to visit her if it is not safe.

Doctor: Oh I see. Well rest assured, the rash is not contagious. When is your daughter expecting?

Patient: Not until next year.

Doctor: I see. Is there anything else I can help you with today?

Patient: Something for the itching?

Doctor: Oh yes. Well the choices are calamine lotion, a mild steroid cream and/or an antihistamine tablet. Which do you prefer? **(PC12, 13)**

Patient: I've got calamine at home. Could I have the other two?

Doctor: Sure.

(Doctor prints off prescription.)

Doctor: Now here's your prescription. You apply the hydrocortisone cream to the rash twice daily as needed, and you can take the antihistamine tablet Piriton four hourly as needed. The rash should clear in a few days. Any questions? **(PC11, 13, 14)**

Patient: No that's fine doctor. Thank you very much.

Doctor: Goodbye.

Transcript of Consultation Reference 6

Child with fever symptoms and a history of vesicoureteric reflux

Doctor: Hello, how can I help you today, Victoria? Go sit on mummy's lap. **(PC1)**

(Greet patient with an engaging smile. The camera should show both the mother and child, so getting the child to sit on mother's lap is one useful tool.

Patient's mother: Right. Victoria has a kidney problem ... recurrent kidney infections. She's had lots of surgeries. She's been on constant antibiotics but was taken off it recently. She told me she was fine but she hasn't been. She's had an infection for the past couple of weeks. She told me she didn't want to go to the hospital. And we don't have any more antibiotics.

Doctor: Oh dear Victoria. So you have been suffering. **(PC2)**

Patient's mother: So she's been suffering. So now she has run out of antibiotics, she's been worse.

Doctor: Is she running a fever? **(PC5)**

Patient's mother: She has been on and off.

Doctor: Can I give you a cup? Can you make wee wee for me? **(PC6)**

Patient's mother: We can try.

(Do not turn off the camera when they exit the room. It's a good time to be seen checking the computer records and filling out the microbiology request form. Fingers crossed they don't take more than 5 minutes.)

Doctor: You're back. Oh that's plenty. Have a seat there please.

(Dipstick the urine or run it on diagnostic machine.) **(PC6)**

Doctor: We'll let that run on the machine there. Now let's check you over. **(PC6)**

(Take temperature, ENT exam, listen to chest.)

Doctor: 37, okay. Everything checks out fine so far. **(PC8)** Now I've noticed on the screen that she hasn't had her meningitis C vaccine? (Health promotion)

Patient's mother: No, she hasn't had it. She was away when they were giving it out.

Doctor: Oh right. Can I make an appointment for her? Next Friday, 9:30?

Patient's mother: 9:30's good. (She is seen writing this in her diary.)

(Machine results print off.)

Doctor: There are a couple of options based on the result. The results show that she may not have an infection this time. The test for infection, nitrates, is clear. There is also no blood in her wee. There are a few white cells, which means there might be a little bit of inflammation. I've noticed on the screen that her last urines have come back normal. Because of her kidney problem, I can give her a prescription now or wait for the lab results next week. What do you think? **(PC7, 8, 9, 10, 11, 12, 13)**

Patient's mother: Can we put her back on her night-time antibiotics and wait and see what that says? Don't want her to have too much antibiotics.

Doctor: That's fine.

(While the printer is printing, take this opportunity to develop rapport with the child.)

Doctor: How's school Victoria? **(PC3)**

Patient (7 years old, F): Okay.

Doctor: What year are you in at school?

Patient: Year 3.

Doctor: Do they give you homework in year 3? They do?

Patient: Well I'm used to it, because we got it in year 2.

Doctor: Oh so you're a big girl already.

Patient's mother: They're saying at school she's not been herself. She's very tired.

Doctor: I see. Is she seeing anyone at the hospital? **(PC2)**

Patient's mother: Yes, every 6 months, Dr X. We see her sooner if she has any positive infections.

Doctor: Has the night-time dose been altered as she is getting older?

Patient's mother: No, she's always been getting the 5 ml dose.

Doctor: Let me check the dose as she is 7 now. On the scales please ... 25 kg. Yes, she's on the right dose. It should be twice her weight, so she's on the correct dose. **(PC13)**

Patient's mother: We had a parent's meeting and the teacher says she's constantly tired.

Doctor: Well, she is running a slight temperature. Do you have any Calpol? **(PC2)**

Patient's mother: No.

Doctor: Let's add paracetamol then.

Patient's mother: That's lovely. Thanks very much.

Doctor: She can take 1 or 2 teaspoons of the paracetamol up to 4 times a day and that's her night-time antibiotics. If you drop the urine bag in the box at reception it will just make pickup. And if you make an appointment for next week, we'll have the results of her urine for you.   (PC14)

Patient's mother: Lovely. Thanks very much.   (PC15)

Transcript of Consultation Reference 7

Heroin drug addiction

Doctor: Hello. How can I help you today? (PC1)

Patient (34 years old, M): I'm here for my scripts for methadone and diazepam.

(Now ideally, repeat prescriptions and follow-up visits should not be used for the video module but here I have included this one as it highlights a social case and you will need to include one meaty psychosocial case – depression, drug addiction, indigent, refugee, etc.)

Doctor: Okay. Last time we started you on 20 ml of methadone. Are you happy with that dose? Are you withdrawing? Are you having to use on top? (PC4, 5)

Patient: I've used once on top in 2 weeks, because I got some money from social security. I've been tempted. I know I've got to deal with that.

Doctor: And when you used that one time did you smoke or inject the heroin? (PC5)

Patient: No just smoked in a roll-up.

Doctor: Okay. Now the last time I saw you I gave you your first hepatitis vaccine, so you're not due for your next one for...   (Health promotion)

Patient: 2 weeks.

Doctor: Exactly, very good, so I'll give you that next time. Now did you have a chance to see the nurse about getting your blood tests?

Patient: No I've been working for the last 12 days, been doing some painting to get some money. I've got the form in the plastic bag, so I will get that done in the next 2 weeks before I see you.

Doctor: And so you know you're being tested for hepatitis b and c? (PC4)

Patient: Yeah.

Doctor: Will you be getting more work painting?

Patient: As some of my friends are painters. They're not drug users. They said I'll give you a chance but you better not mess it up.

Doctor: They're giving you a chance. Good. And what about your living accommodation? Are you living with people who use? (PC3)

Patient: No I've been living with my mum. But they're basically trying to sort me out a hostel, but they're saying they don't want to put me in a hostel because of the risk of drug using in the hostel. They'd rather me go to a bed and breakfast. I've been down to X road but they weren't much help because they're saying that unless you've got a child … But my child is in care. Like they're saying I'm not vulnerable enough, you know what I mean. My mum's putting up with me for now.

Doctor: And how are you putting up with mum? (PC3)

Patient: Yeah, not too bad.

Doctor: Are you getting square meals?

Patient: Yeah that's the thing you know what I mean. I pay my tenner a month and get three meals a day mate.

Doctor: And how's your mood? How are your spirits? (PC3)

Patient: A couple of times I get a bit down. But that's just like, that's what I've got to deal with myself. That's like with the boredom and not having a job and like not being able to see anyone 'cause most of my friends do drugs. So it takes a long time and it's adjusting to that.

Doctor: You are very motivated. (PC2)

Patient: Yeah, I see my parole officer once a week. Have a cup of coffee and chat with them.

Doctor: Do you drink alcohol or smoke cigarettes? (Health promotion)

Patient: Now I ain't being funny but since I've been out of prison, the couple of days I've had a few cans of cider, I've been sick afterwards. So I haven't really drunk. The couple of times I've used it hasn't been the gear that's made me sick, it's been the drink. I used to drink strong lager. I don't even like the alcohol. The times before it was the buzz.

Doctor: What about cigarettes? (Health promotion)

Patient: No, I smoke roll-ups three times a day. You can leave it in the tray and go back to it. Too dear for cigarettes.

Doctor: Have you thought about cutting down on the roll-ups?

Patient: I only smoke three, and if I bought cigarettes I'd be smoking fifteen.

Doctor: I checked your urine result, as we like to check and see if you are taking your methadone. And it does show that you are, but it also picked up a bit of opiates. You had said you topped up once. (PC8, 9)

Patient: Yeah.

Doctor: How do you feel about coming down off the methadone? You're only on 20 ml of methadone. The options are we leave you on 20 ml until you supply a clean urine or we cut down from today by 2 ml a week. How do you feel about that? (PC11, 12, 13)

Patient: Yeah I don't want to get addicted to methadone. Before I was on 30s, 40s 50s and that's worse than the gear you know what I mean.

Doctor: Can you supply a clean urine today? (PC6)

Patient: Yeah think so.

Doctor: Good then let's do that. I'll give you 20 ml for 2 weeks and then next time I see you, you can tell me if you still want to come down. We can go down by 2 ml a week. We'll have a nice clean urine on the screen by then. How do you feel about that?' **(PC11, 12)**

Patient: Yeah that's good.

Doctor: There you are then. See you shortly. (Give urine pot.)

(Keep filming while the patient is absent.)

Patient: I forgot to mention. I need another sick note. My last one was for 6 weeks.

Doctor: Sure. (Drug dependence is a valid reason for an extended med3 cert up to 13 weeks at a time.)

Doctor: Now you're taking diazepam 10 mg/day. I just need to warn you that taken with methadone and with alcohol, it can make you drowsy. Are you driving? **(PC13)**

Patient: No.

Doctor: Because you've been taking diazepam for many, many years, we are going to continue that. If you feel you are ready to come off, we can reduce it. **(PC12, 13)**

Patient: How am I going to reduce diazepam though? Can't be coming down by 5s.

Doctor: No we can go down by 1 mg.

Patient: Can we do that today?

Doctor: Yes. So today, I'll give you a script for 9 mg. Next time I see you, if that's okay we'll go down to 8 mg/day. **(PC12, 13)**

(Print off prescription for diazepam and hand-write methadone on a blue form.)

Doctor: Now I've put Saturday's and Sunday's doses for Friday pick up. You have been taking your methadone, so I am making it easier for you. (reward)

Patient: Oh thanks yeah B closes at noon on Saturdays, and I've been running to the chemist to make it. So now I can go shopping with my mum and that in the mornings.

Doctor: Now if this urine comes back clean, I can go from daily pickups to twice weekly pickups, so there are bonuses. OK here you go, and I'll see you in 2 weeks for your vaccinations and next script. **(PC12, 14)**

Patient: Thanks a lot yeah. **(PC15)**

Transcript of Consultation Reference 8

Dizziness
Headache

Doctor: How can I help you this morning? (PC1)

Patient (51 years old, F): When I came to see the doctor last, she took me off hormone replacement therapy (HRT) because I had a heart attack. About a week ago, I started feeling dizzy but that's one of the reasons why I went on the HRT so I thought it was coming off it. Unfortunately since then I've had this pressure (pointing to the top of her head). It's not a migraine. It's like something is pushing the top of my head. My ears are very sensitive, especially this one (pointing to left ear), and my throat's started to be sore. So I don't know if I've got some sort of virus in my head?

Doctor: It could be. (PC4)

Patient: I haven't had a cough or cold or anything like that. But I just sort of feel like I've been out drinking all night long, and I've got the after effect. But I just don't seem to be there. But my ears just seem to be very, very sensitive.

Doctor: Is anybody else sick at home? (PC5)

Patient: My daughter has been feeling sort of sick. But when she's on antidepressants, I suppose that sometimes gives you that sort of reaction anyways. So apart from that no.

Doctor: How is it affecting your life? Are you at home? (PC3)

Patient: I'm unemployed. But just going out sort of the sun in my face would really make my head hurt but it's only literally in the last week.

Doctor: OK.

Patient: So now my throat is starting to hurt. So there is something definitely wrong.

Doctor: Is it keeping you up at night? (PC5)

Patient: No but when I do reading ... reading is one of my hobbies, I can only read for half an hour, and then I put the book down because my head is just hurting. Something's making my head so sensitive.

Doctor: Is there anything else going on in your life? Any cause for stress? (PC3)

(The doctor here is trying to elicit a cue for PC2. It is a good question to ask and especially if the patient admits to stress as a factor.)

Patient: No. I've learned to deal with stress having a heart attack. That's one of the things you have to learn to deal with. Where as before I used to get frustrated, now I just walk away. When my daughter starts, because she gets moody on antidepressants, I don't argue with her. If anything I am quite calm now than I have been for a long, long time. But as I say it's just been this last week. I feel hot in myself, and it's this ear.

Doctor: How long had you been on the HRT?

Patient: Three or five years. Dr X said to come off it. I only have one day of period if that. Sometimes it's nothing.

Doctor: Shall I check your blood pressure? (PC6)

Patient: Ahem.

(It looks better to be seen using the manual sphygmomanometer.)

Doctor: 142 over 90. That's not bad.

Patient: My teeth in the back here (pointing to her maxilla) are aching too, but I'm not allowed penicillin.

Doctor: Oh, I see. OK, now let's look in your ear. Now is it hurting inside or on the outside of the ear? (PC6)

Patient: It was on the inside but now it's actually going down the back where your pipework goes.

(Doctor is seen examining the ear with an otoscope.)

Doctor: Well that explains it. Your ear is full of wax. It's completely blocked your ear. This might affect your balance and your hearing. (PC7, 8)

Patient: Would that also affect my teeth as well?

Doctor: Well let me continue examining you. Now the other ear has no wax. The eardrum is nice and pink. (PC8)

Patient: My teeth and my head, it's the whole lot that's hurting.

Doctor: Let me look inside your mouth now. Say 'ah.' (Doctor examines the back teeth and throat, and then is seen palpating the neck for nodes.) (PC6)

Doctor: Follow the light with your eyes. (PC6)

(Doctor is seen checking the pupils for reactivity, symmetry, nystagmus, extraocular movements, and photophobia.)

Doctor: I think it is viral as you think too. For the ear, you can either use warm olive oil to soften the wax so it will come out. Because right now your ear is full of wax, and it will make you feel uncomfortable and ... (PC7, 8, 9)

Patient: Affect my balance, yes, hm.

Doctor: and cause dizziness, yes. The other options are using over-the-counter drops like Waxsol or Otex, or I could write you a prescription for sodium bicarb drops, which soften the wax and allows the ear to clean itself out. That might help the ear pain. Now looking at your throat, it's nice and pink. There are no obvious sign of infection right now. Your tonsils are a bit big but still pink. It could be a virus starting to flare up in your throat. (PC8, 9)

Patient: Yes it's just got to my throat last night and this morning.

Doctor: Have you taken anything for the pain?

Patient: Paracetamol because my head has been so muzzy and aching. But I'd rather work through something than take a pill, because I take so many for my heart. I try not to take too many. But as I say this headache is like somebody trying to push me into the floor.

Doctor: Pressure, lots of pressure, yes. Did the paracetamol help?

Patient: It takes the edge off of it but it's not getting rid of it.

Doctor: I can give you ibrufen? Do you have asthma? (PC13)

Patient: Yes, I'm asthmatic.

Doctor: I see. How about something stronger with codeine perhaps? (PC12–13)

Patient: I've had co-codamol. I think that's got codeine in it.

Doctor: Did that help?

Patient: Yes it did help.

Doctor: You didn't get constipated, nauseous?

Patient: Well I've got irritable bowel syndrome (IBS) anyway so I never know from one day to another what I'll be anyway so …

Doctor: Oh right. OK let's give you that then?

Patient: Do I need antibiotics or not? (Patient's real agenda.)

Doctor: I think it is early days now. Shall we see how it goes? Looking at the back of the throat, it is not red or angry. And your ears look fine except for wax in your left ear. Do you want some ear drops?(PC12–13)

Patient: I'll try.

Doctor: Now for the cocodamol, because you have a sore throat, I can give it to you in dispersible form or can you still swallow tablets? (PC13, 14)

Patient: I swallow six tablets in the morning anyway. I take them for the heart and for my cholesterol. But my cholesterol is OK. It's 4.1.

Doctor: Oh that's a very good cholesterol.

Patient: Yeah, people think that because you are big you're unhealthy. But I'm not. My husband before he died was diabetic, so I've kept the kids on low sugar and low fat. So I just automatically buy low fat, sunflower.

Doctor: That is good.

Patient: So when I had my heart attack, I started buying virgin oil.

Doctor: Oh virgin oil is very good.

(Doctor prints off prescriptions.)

Doctor: OK. So you know that because you're taking a painkiller with codeine, it might make you drowsy. Especially important if you are driving. Don't mix it with alcohol. For some people it may cause nausea and constipation. So those are things you should look out for. **(PC13)**

Patient: Okay.

Doctor: Now for your drops. Apply it into your ear up to three times a day. It will soften the wax, and you will start to see wax at the edges of your ear, coming out. It takes a few days, so do use the drops for at least a week. (Doctor hands over prescriptions.) **(PC13)**

Patient: Can I use your scales? I'm normally about 16 and a half.

Doctor: Yes, go ahead.

Patient: Oh my god, I've gone up to 17. I don't believe it.

Doctor: Well we'll keep an eye on it. What sort of things have you been eating?

Patient: Well whereas my sister has been on a diet, I have been eating healthy. So I haven't been eating stir fries. I was 3 weeks on weight watchers and only lost a pound.

Doctor: Well you are trying.

Patient: Yes, I suppose I am. Thank you doctor.

Doctor: Goodbye.

Transcript of Consultation Reference 9

Bilateral breast pain
Back pain
Repeat oral contraception

Doctor: How can I help you today? (PC1)

Patient (19 years old, F): First thing I need a repeat prescription for my pill. Next thing I've been getting really bad pains across this part of my chest (pointing to upper outer quadrant of right breast)…both sides but mainly this side…

(Ah the all too familiar patient with a list. Do not look flustered. Listen to the patient's list calmly and in your mind reflect as to how many items you can safely manage in 15 minutes. If you think you can manage all three, fine, but if not, say to the patient that she has booked a 15-minute appointment, and you will only be able to attend to two items at this consultation. Perhaps ask her to select the most important two. If she becomes hostile, do not take it personally. Be firm. Understand that the patient has unreal expectations of you. This is one tip for time-keeping to 10 minutes in the future and to prevent burnout.)

Doctor: And what did you think was going on? (PC4)

Patient: At first I thought it was a bit of sympathy pains because my best friend was breast-feeding, because I did get swollen ankles and all that when my friend got it. But it's actually got worse. And I've been checking and I couldn't find anything myself, so that's one. And the other thing is I actually done my back in a while ago, and I fell over on the weekend, and I hurt it again. But it's got really bad this time …

Doctor: What do you do for a living? (PC3)

Patient: I work with children. So it's the lifting that hurts. But I could be standing up and feel ooh that's a bit uncomfortable.

Doctor: Yes, okay then. Let's start from the top with your blood pressure and weight.

(The doctor has decided to take on the challenge of all three items on her list in 15 minutes. The doctor is seen using a manual sphygmomanometer with a large cuff to take the patient's blood pressure.) (PC6)

Doctor: Which tablet are you taking?

Patient: It's Cilest.

Doctor: Your blood pressure is 114 over 70. Normal. Now if you can pop on the scale for me please.

(Repeat prescriptions for the pill should not be used as your main consultation video as you will not receive marks. Here marks will be obtained only for the management of both the breast and back pain, which can have serious consequences.)

Doctor: 80 kilos. I'll plug in those numbers and work out your body mass index. It's 34. Now we like to see the number below 30.

Patient: Yeah well I've just come back from holiday.

Doctor: I see. You've been indulging yourself?

Patient: Yeah.

Doctor: Your ideal weight is 54 kilos. If you can try to eat low-fat foods and take up exercise, that would be good. Do you smoke?

Patient: No.

Doctor: Do you drink alcohol?

Patient: Since my friend's been pregnant for the last 9 months, we haven't.

Doctor: Oh you've been very good. Now any headaches or migraines on the pill? **(PC15)**

Patient: No.

Doctor: Okay I can go ahead and issue you a repeat prescription for Cilest but let me check your breasts first. Now if you pop behind the curtain, I can examine your breasts, if that's OK?'

(Be seen to be asking for consent to an intimate examination – breast, rectal, pelvic, etc. Doctor guides patient off camera to the examining couch and draws the curtains. Keep the camera rolling as the examiners will be listening to your dialogue with the patient.)

Doctor: Have you noticed anything different about your breasts? Any lumps? Any nipple discharge? **(PC5)**

Patient: No, nothing at all.

Doctor: Does breast cancer or breast problems run in your family? Mother, sister, aunts on your mother's side, grandmother? **(PC5)**

Patient: No.

Doctor: Have you taken anything for the pain?

Patient: No, 'cause it hasn't been severe …

(Doctor is heard examining the patient's breasts.) **(PC6)**

Doctor: Have you changed your bra recently? Does the pain come during certain times of the month?

Patient: No.

Doctor: There are no breast lumps. Your breast exam is normal. **(PC7, 8)** Now while you're up on the couch, let's examine your back, if that's OK? Can you show me where it hurts? Does the back pain go anywhere?

(PC5)

Patient: It starts at me back and then it sometimes moves up to my neck. Then my neck goes numb. I could smack the back of my neck, and I couldn't feel anything. So I mean I don't know whether it has anything to do with the back or it's me being you know a bit …

Doctor: Alright then. Lie on your back please. I'm just going to raise your legs, so just relax. Any pain when I do this? (dorsiflexing the foot) Any tingling, numbness or weakness in your legs?

Patient: I have actually got weak ligaments.

Doctor: In your knees?

Patient: The doctor says I've got it all over.

Doctor: Can you feel me touching your legs? Is it roughly about the same? And here too and here? Now I'm just going to check your reflexes. Okay, you can take a seat now.

Doctor: What have you been taking for your back pain?

Patient: Nothing. It's there say one day and the next day, I think, um it's not so bad. But while I was on holiday when I actually fell down the stairs while I was away, I did take some painkillers because it was agony. And being on holiday, you don't want to spoil your holiday and go to hospital. So I thought I'd just sit back and keep cool about it. But now that I've come back, it's sort of niggling.

Doctor: I see. Now what you have is called simple or mechanical back pain. **(PC7, 8, 11, 12)** Now what happens is that the muscles in your back go into spasm, and then you stiffen, get sore and get back pain. The treatment options are taking painkillers such as ibuprofen or paracetamol to start with and stronger ones if necessary or using back-strengthening exercise such as when you lie on your back, lift your legs up together so you can feel the pressure in your back as you strengthen the muscles. Also use good posture techniques, bend at your knees and not your back when you lift a child up. Does that make sense? **(PC10)**

Patient: Yes.

Doctor: I can also print out a help sheet for you for back pain if you like.

Patient: Yes.

Doctor: Now what would you like to do? Would you like me to give you painkillers or would you like to try the exercises? **(PC12, 13)**

Patient: Um, if I try the exercises and see how it goes. If not, I can always take a paracetamol.

Doctor: Now with the pain in your breasts, I've checked you out for lumps because we just want to make sure that there is nothing bad there. Now with breast pain, the treatments are paracetamol, evening primrose oil or a special stronger medication that I need to prescribe. So which would you like to try? **(PC8, 9, 11–13)**

Patient: I'll just see how it goes. I can take a paracetamol if it bothers me.

Doctor: Okay let me give you your prescription for Cilest. Do you have a booklet on the pill at home?

Patient: No.

Doctor: Would you like one? It tells you what to do if you take antibiotics, have diarrhoea, miss a pill and you don't know what to do. It's good to have it handy.

Patient: Many a times have I missed a pill.

Doctor: Oh dear. It is hard to remember sometimes. Any problems with that? (PC2)

Patient: No, luckily.

Doctor: Now let me print off the help sheet on back pain. They used to say bedrest was the treatment, but now they've discovered that actually strengthening the back is better so the muscles can support your back. Also losing weight is a good idea as there will be less weight for your back to support. Why don't you get the children at the nursery to do your exercises with you? (PC9)

Patient: Yes, good idea. They would love that.

Doctor: Excellent. Here are the pages for you to read and it includes some of those back exercises too. And if the back pain persists for more than 2 weeks, do come back and see me. (PC14)

Patient: Thank you, I will.

Transcript of Consultation Reference 10

Foot pain
Vertigo

Doctor: How can I help you today? (PC1)

Patient (52 years old, M): Things have come undone underneath and it's really stinging me.

Doctor: How is it affecting you day to day? (PC3)

Patient: Well with my job I do a lot of walking and that. It really hurts. Let me show you. (Patient removes his shoes.)

Doctor: What have you used?

Patient: Cream.

Doctor: Has it helped?

Patient: Yeah. See this, look at the state of my feet. That bit's the cream I put on it. It's just getting worse and worse.

Doctor: Yes, it's athlete's foot with the flaking and the cracking of the skin.

Patient: Especially between the toes, they're splitting. Some of them are really painful at times.

(Doctor is thinking there must be a hidden agenda. Athlete's foot must be his calling card. For video consultation purposes, make sure that the main problem is not athlete's foot as this has no serious implications and you may fail on grounds of poor choice of cases.)

Doctor: Anything else going on? (PC2)

Patient: Yeah, there's something wrong with my right ear. I've been getting vertigo.

Doctor: When you say vertigo, do you mean that the room was spinning or you felt unsteady on your feet like on a ship? (PC4)

Patient: Unsteady like. I get it now and again, not on a regular basis. Last couple of days I've been getting it more.

Doctor: Have you had your blood pressure checked recently? (PC5)

Patient: Yeah.

Doctor: Was that alright?

Patient: Yeah, not high, nothing like that.

Doctor: And what do you think is going on? (PC4)

Patient: I think it could be to do with the right ear.

Doctor: What do you mean by the right ear?

Patient: If I'm laying down on my right ear and I move, suddenly I go giddy. If I do it the other way, I don't go giddy.

Doctor: So it's positional. (PC2)

Patient: Yeah. Now and again I get up and feel ooh a bit giddy.

Doctor: Do you have any problems with your hearing? Do you get ringing in your ears? (PC5)

Patient: No, nothing like that.

Doctor: Have you ever been exposed to loud noise, gunfire, loud music? What kind of work do you do? (PC3)

Patient: I do drive a loud diesel machine. It's a sweeping machine I walk along with.

Doctor: And how long have you been doing this job?

Patient: Ooh, quite a few years, 5 or 6 years now.

Doctor: Have you ever asked anyone to repeat themselves in conversations?

Patient: Not really, unless they are really quiet talking and then I might say sorry or excuse me.

Doctor: Right. Shall I look in your ear then? (PC6)

Patient: Yep.

(The doctor is seen examining the ears with an otoscope. Always examine the 'good' ear first.)

Doctor: There's a fair amount of wax in your left ear. (PC7, 8)

Patient: Yeah I try to clean it out as best I can.

Doctor: What do you use?

Patient: I just normally get a cotton bud to try to get it out. But I don't like to do it too much as it makes me feel sick.

Doctor: Okay your right ear looks fine, but the left ear is full of wax. Now cotton buds to clean out the ears are not advised. What happens is that the cotton bud ends up pushing some of the wax up against your eardrum and it gets stuck there. And then you're not getting the right input to your ear and your balance goes. Does that make sense?' (PC8, 10)

Patient: Yup, yup.

Doctor: Now the treatment options are you can either use warmed up olive oil at home to soften the wax or drops over the counter such as Waxsol or Otex, or I can give you a prescription for sodium bicarb drops. (PC11, 13) The drops will soften the wax and then the ear cleans itself out so you don't have to clean the ear. It's a normal process where the skin of the inside of the ear is always moving outwards, and it takes the wax with it out of your ear. But if you use cotton buds, you interrupt that process and the wax gets stuck.

Patient: Oh I see what you mean.

Doctor: And it does make you lightheaded and dizzy when you have impacted wax in your ear.

Patient: Yeah and I've been getting sick and all.

Doctor: Yes.

Patient: I mean if I go on a boat I get sea-sick.

Doctor: Oh so you are sensitive. Now your right ear looks normal, the ear-drum and the ear canal. So that's something to think about and may be the cause of your dizziness. Now what would you like to do?

(PC12)

Patient: Yeah, if you could advise some drops perhaps I could try them?

Doctor: Yes, absolutely. Now if you use the drops and still have wax, then you can see the nurse for ear syringing too. If your ears ever feel itchy, then come back for different drops, because that means the lining of your ears are irritated. Don't poke or scratch the inside of your ears …

Patient: Oh yeah and make it worse.

Doctor: Exactly. Okay so let me print you off your two prescriptions.

Patient: Sometimes if I take the sea-sickness pills it makes the giddiness go away.

Doctor: Now with the sea-sickness pills, they are like a sedative. They calm down your inner ear, which controls balance so then your inner ear is not working. So what you should be doing is exercises to train your inner ear to get used to different positions and not feeling sick. It's like going on a roller coaster or being an ice-skater. You do it in stages other-wise everyone would get dizzy doing that.

(Doctor is trying to explain that exercises can habituate vertigo.)

Patient: Yeah that's right.

Doctor: So if your dizziness gets really bad, then take the pills for a few days but don't rely on it all the time. Now this prescription is for your feet. It's an anti-fungal cream. Use it three times a day and continue using it 2 weeks after the infection has cleared. You also need to apply it to the normal surrounding skin too.

(PC13)

Would you like a help sheet on things you can do to prevent getting athlete's foot?

Patient: Yeah.

(Doctor prints off help sheet and second prescription.)

Doctor: Here is the prescription for the ear drops. Apply the drops four times a day to your left ear for at least a week. Now let me go through the help sheet with you. It's very common. One in ten people get it. It's a little fungus that likes to live in skin, especially in moist areas and your job entails a lot of walking you said ... (Patient is seen reading the sheet with the doctor.) (PC11, 13)

Patient: Yeah my feet do get sweaty, walking about all day driving that machine, and now it's just gradually got worse.

Doctor: Yes, I see that. Here are your prescriptions. Now if the dizziness persists for more than 2 weeks, do come back and see me. (PC14)

(Doctor hands over the script and help sheet to the patient.)

Patient: Okay, lovely. Thanks very much.

Doctor: You're welcome. Bye bye.

Transcript of Consultation Reference 11

'Bad chest'
'Terrible cold'

Doctor: How can I help you today? (PC1)

Patient (67 years old, F, heavy smoker): Well, I've got a terrible cold and I've got a bad chest and I went in last year to hospital with a chest infection. So I thought I must come in and see you and get something to help me with the chest because I don't want to go into hospital.

Doctor: Yes indeed. Are you coughing up anything? (PC5)

Patient: No, nothing comes up at all.

Doctor: Do you smoke? (PC5)

Patient: I do. But I've been trying to leave it off a bit while I've got this bad chest.

Doctor: And how many cigarettes do you smoke in a day?

Patient: Oh about 20 in a day.

Doctor: And for how long?

Patient: Oh long time. Ever since I was young.

Doctor: How often do you get these chest infections?

Patient: I don't get them all the time. It seems when the weather gets damp and cold.

Doctor: About once a year?

Patient: Yeah, usually.

Doctor: Are you running a temperature? (PC5)

Patient: Oh I don't know really.

Doctor: Any sweating at night? (PC5)

Patient: Oh sweating. Yeah, I wake up in the morning sweating.

Doctor: Have you lost any weight? (PC5)

Patient: Oh I've been losing weight for a long time 'cause I've got a gullet problem and an intestine problem. I attend the hospital for it and I have pills for it, special pills. And that causes me I can't eat properly 'cause it catches in the gullet. So I have to be careful of what I eat. So I eat all soft foods. Yeah I have a problem there.

Doctor: Do you have any other problems like diarrhoea or constipation? (PC5)

Patient: No.

Doctor: It's just with food going down?

Patient: Yeah, just the food.

Doctor: And what is going on in your life? (PC3)

Patient: Oh everything's fine at the moment. As a matter of fact I'm going to Spain at the end of the month. I'm moving out there.

Doctor: You're moving to Spain!

Patient: Yeah, so that's why I don't want this (pointing to her chest).

Doctor: No, you're not going to get it over there with lots of sunshine. No cold weather. (PC2)

Patient: No.

Doctor: Do you have family or are you going by yourself?

Patient: No, I'm going with my partner.

Doctor: With your partner.

Patient: And um, I hope it will be nice. Me family's coming out to see me in May.

Doctor: Oh excellent, so you won't lose touch.

Patient: Oh no. There's four of them so they'll all be out there.

Doctor: Oh big reunion. So tell me about your chest infection. When did it start?

Patient: Two years ago.

Doctor: No, I mean this recent one.

Patient: Well, last year I had to go into hospital and they put me on a drip. They said I was anaemic so I've been taking these iron pills all the time. You know I have them every day, three or four times a day to keep my bloods and vitamins you know. I still seem to have caught it though. So I was wondering whether you could give me something.

Doctor: Yes. I'd like to examine you now. I'd also like to check your blood pressure if I may, because you said you were anaemic. (PC6)

Patient: I've been taking my pills regular. So I should be alright.

Doctor: Have you had your flu jab this year? (Health promotion)

Patient: No, I haven't had it and I was gonna ask you if I could still have it with this cold you know.

Doctor: Oh I see. Yes, you might have to wait a week until you are better.

Doctor: Have you ever had a chest x-ray? (PC5)

Patient: I can't remember.

Doctor: When you were in hospital last year perhaps?

Patient: They might have done.

Doctor: Have you had an x-ray this year?

Patient: No, I don't think so. But I have been getting breathless and all that you know.

Doctor: Yes, it's difficult for you.

(Doctor is seen changing the cuff to a small cuff and using a manual sphygmomanometer to take patient's blood pressure.)

Doctor: 150 over 78. Your blood pressure is a tad up. I'll look and see what your blood pressure has been running.

(Doctor checks computer screen.)

Doctor: Actually you had a blood test in May that showed you weren't anaemic, so that's good. It shows that your iron is working.   (PC9)

Patient: I had to have a blood transfusion when I was in the hospital last year. My blood got that low. All night long they was doing it.

Doctor: Oh right. Now your blood pressure has come down since January.

Patient: Oh good. So the pills are doing me good then.

Doctor: Yes. So we'll carry on with that.

Patient: So there's nothing wrong with me blood?

Doctor: No, you've got enough blood in you. Let me listen to your chest now if I may. Could you stand up for me please, and I'll just slip the stethoscope under your top from behind. Now breathe in and out through your mouth please.   (PC6)

(Always ask the patient to stand when auscultating the chest or asking the patient to use a peak flow meter.)

Doctor: Have a seat there. You're not getting good air flow through your lungs. I'd agree with you regarding your chest infection. Shall I weigh you? I just want to keep an eye on your weight loss.   (PC7, 8, 9)

(Patient gets on scale.)

Doctor: 55 kilos. Have a seat again. I'll plug those numbers in. Actually your weight has come up a bit since January. Now that is good. And before you were a bit underweight, but now you are perfect for your height and weight. (Patient smiles.)

Patient: Is this the right weight?

Doctor: Yes.

Patient: Good.

Doctor: Now about your smoking. Have you thought about the patches or are you just not ready? (Health promotion)

Patient: Not ready. See I have a nerve problem that's why I smoke.

Doctor: What do you mean by a nerve problem? (PC4)

Patient: Well I suffer from me nerves. I go down to see the doctor in the hospital every 3 months for me nerves.

(Doctor looks baffled.)

Doctor: Nerves?

Patient: Well I used to get what they call illusions you know.

Doctor: Did you hear things or see things?

Patient: Hear. I used to hear voices (pointing to her temple).

Doctor: Did they put you on medication?

Patient: Oh yeah.

Doctor: And you've been on it for a while?

Patient: Oh yeah. Few years now.

Doctor: So have the voices settled down? Do you hear voices now?

Patient: Oh no. I'm fine now.

(Patient starts hacking.)

Doctor: Oh dear you do have a bad cough. Well, we'll give you antibiotics. I think that's the only option here. I don't think we should wait and see. I don't think you'll get better. What do you think? (PC7, 8, 12, 13)

Patient: No, I do need help. It's been going on for 3 weeks.

Doctor: Why did you wait 3 weeks?

Patient: Well I thought it would go. I kept saying I can't bother the doctor and in the end I thought I'd better go to the doctors.

Doctor: I'd like to give you a week of antibiotics. If it doesn't clear up, then I'd like to arrange a chest x-ray because with you smoking, the smoking can cause a bit of damage to your chest. Does that sound like a good plan? (PC12, 14)

Patient: Yeah, very good.

Doctor: Now are you allergic to any medicines that I should know about? (PC13)

Patient: No. They should be alright with my medicines because I have had antibiotics before.

Doctor: Yes, that's fine. I'm going to give you a strong dose.

Patient: There's nothing I shouldn't be having while taking them?

Doctor: No, I've checked your meds. Now this antibiotic you take three times a day for a week until you finish the bottle. Now what happens if you finish the bottle and it hasn't gone away? (PC11, 13, 14)

Patient: Come down and see you.

Doctor: Yes.

Patient: I will. I promise. I will come back. (Doctor hands over the prescription.)

Patient: Thank you doctor. Thank you very much. (Patient shakes doctor's hand.)